KAPUNA

How Love Transformed a Culture

ERIN FOLEY

Kapuna
How Love Transformed a Culture
By Erin Foley © 2015

For special discounts on print or eBooks, please visit AlohaPublishing.com or email Maryanna@AlohaPublishing.com.

To contact Erin Foley, email eefoley@gmail.com
or visit her blog at speaklifespeakup.wordpress.com

Print ISBN: 978-1-61206-101-6
eBook ISBN: 978-1-61206-109-2

Interior & Cover Design by: Fusion Creative Works, www.fusioncw.com
Editors: Hannah Cross and Manaal Ibrahim
Cover Photo Credit: Gerald Bengessar

Published by

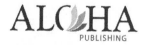

AlohaPublishing.com
Boise, ID

First Edition
Printed in the United States of America

To the people of Papua New Guinea:

No matter where I have been in your beautiful country, you have taken me into your hearts and made me *wantok*. I cannot begin to tell you how much you all have changed my heart and my life. You have an unquenchable strength and beauty.

Dave Weitz
649 S. Woodhaven Ave.
Meridian, ID 83642-3538

"SYMPATHY IS NO SUBSTITUTE FOR ACTION."

– David Livingstone

CONTENTS

INTRODUCTION

Africa.

I am definitely going to Africa.

I pored over maps of Africa, dreaming of the day I would step off a tiny bush plane into the sweltering heat and winds of a remote tribal land somewhere in Africa. Ingrained in me at a young age was the idea that if I wanted to be involved in foreign missions, I would have to go to Africa. I am not even sure where I got the notion.

I can't even recount the number of flyers, pamphlets, and posters I saw that advertised the "needs" and "work" to be done in Africa. From time to time, they showed the face of the African child with a smaller shadow of a South American or Asian child looking out from behind it. On the whole, however, it was a nondescript, skinny African face I remember seeing in my mind.

I had it all planned out. I visualized emerging from a circular hut made of local resources. I would take in a deep breath while people would be squatting over fires in the morning mists, cooking their breakfast—the same plain, starchy breakfast they had the previous morning. Donned in nothing but simple wraps of bright material around chests or midsections, we would chat in a tribal language.

I dreamt of Africa, even sponsored a child from Africa. If I was not living in it as a missionary, I'd be a foreign correspondent who traveled there, writing harrowing tales of civil wars and tribal clashes.

Yet, here I was on a bush plane flying over the lush, river-veined terrain of the Melanesian island of Papua.

At thirty-one years old, I still have never been to Africa.

As we ascended from the tarmac, I watched as the city faded below. The last few glimpses of Port Moresby gave way to the incredible azure of the ocean and a rugged, green coastline. It was my first time sitting at the front of any airplane.

Like most people, my experience was limited to varying sizes of commercial passenger flights, although never any this small and certainly never any where I sat in the copilot seat. On its best day, this aircraft could hold nine passengers and limited cargo. The young pilot from New Zealand gave me a quick smile and then returned his focus to flying. I watched the many dials and instruments and tried to discern what each one was telling me.

Quickly, though, my gaze was drawn out the window. The view was breathtaking. The "Land of the Unexpected" never seemed to disappoint. As a storm front passed, the plane turned to the left and we floated through the last bit of cloud. I watched as it evaporated in the propeller. Our quick ride through the cloud brought us in a northwesterly direction. We would follow the southern coast of Papua New Guinea to a remote area in the Gulf Province.

As I sat gazing, I could tell where the mouth of a river was about to open by the mingling of the muddy river water with the pristine blue of the ocean.

The river systems in PNG are the arteries of life for the island nation. Rivers provide the main supplies of food, drinking and cooking water, a place to bathe, and the key source of transportation. It is by these rivers that life in the Gulf Province exists. It was on one of these tributaries that an incredible story of a bush hospital has been unfolding since the 1950s: the story of Kapuna. Little did I know, Kapuna would not only tell an incredible story of hope and life, it would bring me healing, peace, and a family of multiple tribes and tongues.

The tiny plane glided smoothly above the vast bush where the clearing was broken only from time to time by palm-roofed huts.

I was in awe of where my life had taken me these past few years. How on earth did I end up in Papua New Guinea?

The first time I learned anything about Papua New Guinea was in middle school when my sister and I were playing a National Geographic game. There was a dark man on a playing card with bright yellow and red paint smeared across his face, colorful bird plumage engulfed his head, and a pig tusk was hung around his neck. My sister held the card in front of my face.

"Where is it?" Bethany asked.

"Somewhere in Africa? I'm just not sure what area," I responded.

"Wrong!" she said triumphantly flipping the card over, "Papua New Guinea."

"Where's that?"

We searched the giant map on the board game. We were looking in the wrong spot. It took us a while to find the eastern half of the island that floated just above Australia. PNG was not part of my history, geography, or even remotely on my radar for the next decade of my life.

It certainly was not on my list of places to visit in the world.

THE LITTLE WHITE-SKIN

I sat on a hard, wooden bench trying to adjust my blue sundress, crinkled beneath me. Brushing sticky blond curls out of my eyes, I shyly surveyed the little classroom. Dark brown faces with even darker brown, curious eyes peered back at me. Realizing they were all looking at me, I quickly glanced at my feet, pretending I did not notice them.

Being painfully timid at four years old, I hated any form of attention from my peers. On the tiny Caribbean island of Grenada, my fair skin and blond hair did nothing but attract attention. I found out later I was the first white child most of the school children had ever seen. Incredibly conscious of the eyes boring into the back of my head, I watched as my dad and a team of missionaries performed skits and songs for the school. My chubby, sunburned legs swung to the rhythm of the songs I had heard practiced hundreds of times.

I was a missionary kid, also known as a third culture kid. By that age, I had already lived on an old bus that traveled across America, slept on countless church floors or strangers' homes, and my handful of plush animals and toys fit into a small backpack. How could I have known how adept I would become to living out of a suitcase? The only part of this lifestyle I think I never got used to was being stared at for being white . . . not to mention, I was usually also a head taller than the locals. To this day, I wish I could become more of a chameleon.

A year later, my family moved to the sweltering desert town of Monterrey, Mexico. I don't remember much except for the orange dust, maybe some communist signs in Spanish, refried beans with small rocks in them, and the scorpions. Just as in Grenada, my blond hair made me stand out for the foreigner I was. Unlike Grenada, however, it made me more of a target for bullies. My parents worked at a children's home where many of the kids were unwanted and discarded by their families. It did not take long for many of them to turn their hurt and anger on my siblings and me. My sweet, gentle nature was challenged more than once as I faced-off with a group of older girls who picked on my sister. My tanned little fists were clenched as gravel embedded my bleeding knees. They would learn not to push Bethany down again.

It was a moment in my life when I discovered that despite all of my shyness and fear of the world, I would not back down from a fight if it was the right thing to do. I was too young to understand the implications of it all, but I now recognize that it was then that I learned to hate injustice.

Despite my negative impressions from Mexico, I was a child in love with other languages and cultures. Spanish is still one of the most beautiful languages to my ears.

VENEZUELA

At the age of seven, my American childhood remained anything but ordinary. Boarding the overseas flight in Miami, we made our way to Caracas, Venezuela. My parents had hopes of opening a children's home using the knowledge and experience they had gleaned in Mexico. My father had visited barrios outside of Caracas and returned to us determined we would go there to help.

Venezuela was a lesson in the complexities of community development. Not everyone gets on board with a vision, even a positive one. Not everyone is moral; corruption within governments and communities is a huge indirect—and sometimes direct—proponent of poverty.

The journey did not start out well for me. A swollen rash irritated my left leg and I was airsick for most of the flight. Touching down in the South American city, we caught two faded yellow cabs to our new home. Bumper to bumper, car horns blasted while we wove our way through dense traffic. We pulled up to a once affluent neighborhood which now sat barricaded behind metal security gates. Several stair-step levels of the house worked their way up the hill sides.

Our landlady, Francia, had come from a wealthy family but all that remained of her family's inheritance was this large house. She had carved it into a number of small flats, renting them out to ex-patriots in order to make a living. Her friendly face appeared at the gate when we rang the buzzer. Sifting through a fistful of keys, she opened the gate for us and the few duffle bags we carried full of our worldly possessions. Hugs and kisses on both cheeks were exchanged.

The small one bedroom flat off the first terrace was our home. My parents occupied the bedroom while my siblings and I slept on mattresses that pulled out from under a single bed in the lounge room. The flat boasted dusty red brick flooring and barred windows with sheer curtains. We soon found cockroaches and rats also shared our living space.

However, in no time, we made it home. My mother has a knack for turning every dwelling into a home with her special little touches. It always began with scrubbing the place from top to bottom. Daily cleaning was a necessary ritual to combat the grime kicked up from the busy city streets.

These were my earliest memories. These memories shaped me and my future. After my family's plans in Venezuela fell through, we returned to the States, settling into a different kind of life, a life I never fit into. My skin and hair now matched my schoolmates', but my heart never would.

THE CHALLENGE
(YEMBI-YEMBI)

Years later, I was listening to a man who stood on stage with a six-foot-long spear poised in the throwing position. He explained that many people of the tribe in East Sepik, Papua New Guinea, in which he served, had threatened to throw spears if baptisms took place. He had lived in that remote village for five years as a Bible translator with New Tribes Mission and when it came time to baptize the new Christians in the murky, crocodile infested river, many in the tribe were opposed, even to the point of threatening. Eventually the spears of the tribe's people had flown, but every single weapon had missed its mark.

It was the first time I had heard about the nation of Papua New Guinea since the board game with my sister.

That man from Southern California would be a key to God changing my entire world. Tim Shontere had come to my church, The Pursuit, in Boise, Idaho while on his furlough: a year back in the States to reconnect with supporters and family, as well as rest. I sat near the front, completely enthralled as he shared his journey of faith and life as a Bible translator in remote East Sepik, which lies on the northern border of PNG.

I watched his introduction video. A small airplane landed on a grass strip and then a long canoe ride took them into the dense foliage, a lengthy hike and they were in the small village.

It was amazing: The rats, the crocodiles, the infestation of insects, and his challenge to make the Yembi-Yembi tribe a home for his American wife and boys. As enthralled as I was, I sat there knowing there was no way on earth I could live under similar circumstances. Absolutely no way!

Something deep within me stirred at Tim's story. Tears spilled down my face as I listened. I admired people like him who had such faith, who loved God so much they could sacrifice everything—even their life. Fear actually gripped my heart at that moment. What if God were to ask me to do something similar with my life?

I knew I could not. Another emotion emerged: jealousy, but not for his lifestyle so much as a deep jealousy for his *willingness.*

As much as I wanted to be a part of foreign missions, I liked the idea of a home to return to in the States. I had a beautiful apartment that was decorated exactly how I wanted it, full of hard-earned kitchen appliances, furniture, and books. Despite my childhood years in the developing world, I had become comfortable in the first world.

I had life all planned out. I would get a job at a private academy where I would teach art and writing. I would then spend my summers in Africa helping to build houses or loving kids in an orphanage. I would give generously. It would be perfect! I could have the best of both worlds. Wasn't it a worthy pursuit?

Yet, as Tim continued to speak, I knew God did not just want my summer breaks or my generosity. He wanted everything.

I remembered I balled up my fists. I was still holding onto something. Paul, my pastor, had pointed out how many people claimed a willingness to die for God. The harder challenge was not dying for God, but living for God. I was not sure I could do it, but in that moment I knew I had to uncurl my fists, open my hands, and surrender my plans, even my life.

The next few years, everything changed. It was not a harsh or immediate transition, just an unveiling of my true heart. It was a slow, gentle emerging of who I was created to be. As a frustrated young woman who never fit into the American lifestyle, I was on the path to finding out why. By January 2011, I boarded a flight across the world to Australia where I joined a Youth with a Mission (YWAM) team from Townsville.

WAITING AND SUBMITTING

A white dry-erase board was wheeled in front of my Discipleship Training School (DTS) in Townsville, Australia. All 37 of us students waited breathlessly to see what our options for outreach were. Our leader, Naomi, began writing up options as she explained each one.

The first: Papua New Guinea trekking team. This team would train tirelessly to trek some of the hardest terrain in the world, doing village assessments as they went from village to village in the highlands of PNG. Many of these villages were so remote and unknown they did not exist on any map. The trekking team was also going to chart out where each village was, population, access to medical treatment, etc. It was going to be grueling.

My heart almost beat out of my chest when I saw that option. How incredibly awesome! It combined a physical challenge with missions; I was intrigued.

The next option was serving onboard a medical ship in the Gulf Province of PNG, followed by a team that would travel to the Northern Territory to work in aboriginal communities, with another three weeks in the tiny nation of Timor-Leste building houses, and, finally, a team that would travel down the Queensland coast doing youth programs.

I was positive PNG was where I wanted to be.

A few days later, we wrote down our first and second choices on a piece of paper, and handed them into our leaders. Then, we waited.

One evening, I returned from a run, reveling in the tropical birds calling to each other and whiffs of fragrant frangipanis, when Naomi approached me.

"Can I talk to you?" she asked.

Immediately, I knew it was about outreach.

"I would like you to pray and consider not getting your first option for outreach. The staff has been praying and we believe you should consider Timor-Leste. Can you give me your answer in a few days?"

My heart fell.

"Okay," I responded, wanting to find a place to be alone and cry in disappointment for a bit.

Once I was alone, I began to pray. I had not realized how set my heart was on PNG until it was taken away. "God, what do I do?" I asked.

Trust your leaders. Learn to submit. I have a lot to teach you through this.

Until this point in my life, as a single 27-year-old, I was pretty used to making all of my own decisions. I knew God was right. This was not about PNG. This was about me learning to trust and submit to other people, especially leaders.

The next day, I approached Naomi and said, "I trust you as a leader. I prayed and believe I am supposed to be on whatever team you feel is best for me." I was sad, but I knew in my heart this was the right thing.

A few days later, our teams were announced. I was going to the Northern Territory and Timor-Leste. The only part of all of this that left me confused was I still believed Papua New Guinea was in my future, but how and when was unknown.

I am so grateful I said, "Yes," to Timor-Leste. Not only was submission on many levels a valuable lesson in my life, I had an incredible outreach experience. I could not have asked for a better team to have served alongside.

I also found myself completely enthralled with village life. We spent three weeks in a village called Suertulan where we taught English and healthcare, along with building houses. The nation was twelve years into recovery from a brutal genocide at the hands of Indonesia in 1999.

Timor-Leste is a young country exuding hope. I was incredibly encouraged for its future after meeting so many locals who took pride in their nation and sought to build a brighter life. I had my first real taste of developing world village life and I loved it! Despite the rats, squatty potties, and limited resources, I built a dream house in my heart on a mountainside where I might dwell someday. I could definitely see myself living in a village.

That was the shifting point of my life's paradigm. Nine months later, I moved to Australia permanently to work with YWAM Townsville.

THE MEDICAL SHIP: FINALLY, PAPUA NEW GUINEA

On staff with YWAM Townsville and YWAM Medical Ships Australia (YWAM MSA), I worked in the Director's Office. Wearing many hats, the majority of my job revolved around making articles and stories out of the information I received from our medical ship in PNG. I also sorted through the thousands of photos from the returned photographers, editing and organizing.

I used these to keep our website, Facebook page, and newsletters updated. I had one of my dream jobs: writing, content layout, media, photo editor, etc. I was completely captivated with our work on the medical ship. Story after amazing story filtered through me about miracles, amazing medical opportunities, and beautiful faces of volunteers from around the globe.

I was incredibly passionate about our work and what I wrote; the problem was I lacked the firsthand experience. My imagination failed to offer the full scope of experience in remote Papua New Guinea.

August 2012, I was finally going to Papua New Guinea!

Outfitted with camera gear on my back, I boarded the flight to Port Moresby. I was going as the medical ship's media and communications staff. I would spend my days and nights photographing clinics, interviewing, observing, and writing stories.

Looking out of the plane window, I watched the distant lapping waves of the Torres Strait waters. As the flight descended for the landing, I saw the green rolling hills around Port Moresby.

Stepping off the plane, the glaring tropical sun assaulted my eyes. I surveyed my surroundings, taking in the sights and sounds. I wanted to drink it up and remember every second of this experience. I was in PNG, finally!

Entering the Jacksons International Airport from the tarmac, I was immediately met with large, bright colorful faces of different tribal peoples painted on the wall by the visa desk. Paying one hundred kina, the equivalent of about 50 US dollars, my passport received a large yellow sticker with a bird of paradise and a stamp indicating I was permitted 60 days in the country.

A group of the volunteers for the ship gathered around the luggage conveyor belt. Lugging the medical supplies for the ship, as well as our own provisions, we found our friends who were waiting to take us to the ship. Carting the bags outside to the van, I was immediately met with the smell of burning wood and exhaust.

I breathed deeply. It was the scent of a developing world city. Exhaling slowly, I was content. I was home. I wanted to cry with joy.

The crazy hired van ride began. We flew at excessive speeds through crowded streets, circling roundabouts. I thought our van might career onto its side from the momentum. Almost running over pedestrians, our taxi finally made it to the ship yard where the Pacific Link was docked; it was even more exhilarating. I forgot how much I enjoyed the adrenaline pumping traffic in the developing world.

The sidewalks outside of the ship yard were stained bright red from people spitting betel nut (*buai*), a nut that is chewed with lime powder (*kambang*) and a bean-like green called mustard (*daka*), creating a frightfully bright red stain on mouths and teeth. It will eventually break down teeth, rotting them and staining them black.

Had I not been informed of *buai* in Timor-Leste, I would have thought blood was spattered intermittently throughout the streets of Port Moresby.

Needless to say, we made it intact. Donning our safety vests and hard hats, we entered the ship yard. As I walked toward our docked medical ship, I could hardly have predicted just how much my entire world view and life were about to change.

SEASICKNESS AND MUD

The Coral Sea lay before me, an almost unbroken deep blue. As the *M/V Pacific Link* began sailing along Papua New Guinea's southern coast, I sat at the bow in place of a figure-head, my bare feet dangling over the side. The ship dipped so low sometimes, the sea spray and fresh air turned into a blasting wall of salt water. My brown, sun-kissed hair whipped around my face into a knotted mess.

I was drenched but my heart was blissful.

This hunk of whitewashed metal was an old Japanese fishing vessel. After massive overhauls, it found another worthy calling: a medical ship. Outfitted with a crew of fifty, medical supplies crammed in every available corner, and a built-in clinic, the *M/V Pacific Link* made her way to PNG's Western Province. It was on this vessel I would learn the resilience of human nature and find my true calling.

For hours, I sat on the bow. Day turned to night. I was alone but not lonely as it was difficult to be lonely on a small ship packed with crew members. The sun set across the glistening waters, while dolphins followed our boat. I read once that Roman mariners saw dolphins as a good omen and wondered how accurate those statistics were for the ancient sailors.

After about four hours, I reluctantly gave up my spot and blundered across the deck trying to maintain my balance. My sea legs were useless so I clung to the railing. The ship dipped and rolled; ocean spray buffeted me on every side as I fumbled my way to the aft deck and down a steep flight of steps.

The heat of the engine room immediately overwhelmed my senses. With the old vessel traveling around nine knots, the engine room emitted a clamor and sweat-inducing temperatures. It made me nauseous to go from fresh sea air to the enclosed, oily ventilation. I felt a twinge of empathy for the guys working down there, wondering how they survived long sails.

I stumbled past the engine room door just as a large wave rolled the ship to the left. I staggered into a wall with my shoulder. The *M/V Pacific Link* was built for efficiency, not comfort. "Smooth sailing" was a laughable term.

Opening the door I groped my way through the mess hall, along the tables. The stairs to our bunks—located in the belly of the ship—were off the mess hall and galley. As the ship pitched again, I stretched to grab the stair rail before making my final decent.

After stripping off my damp clothes, I put on my pajamas, popped a few seasickness tablets, and crawled into my bunk. We still had over twenty hours to sail.

I soon realized my mistake. The boat constantly rolled, not with a consistent front-to-back or side-to-side motion, but an all-over, unpredictable movement. I lay still with solitary focus. *Do not throw up*, I thought. *Deep breathing*. I tried to ignore my lurching stomach in effort to lull myself to sleep.

I drifted off but awakened a few hours later to the horrendous sound of a crew member gasping and retching. A cold sweat broke out on my brow.

God, help me! I have to get out of here, I prayed.

Determined to escape my dark enclosure, I threw back my blankets. I did a military crawl out of my bunk, stood up, and made a mad dash upstairs. I emerged into the lit mess hall where people were sprawled out on benches or sat with their heads in their hands. At least I was not the only one feeling wretched!

A few people, unaffected by the ship's movements, played cards in a corner and even ate dinner. Though my stomach rebelled, I envied them.

I opened the mess hall door to head toward the bathroom when I smashed my shins on the door jam. The ship's doors are smaller and set higher up, making those on board pick up their legs and duck their heads. I had not remembered this.

Bruises forming, I found the toilet in time to hear a woman vomit in the showers. At least I was not alone.

At this point, my desire to live aboard a ship was erased. Why had I ever thought this was a good idea? I had relished the idea. I had anticipated my life on the *M/V Pacific Link* with absolute elation.

When I had first been told I was going to be the media and communications staff on the *M/V Pacific Link*, I spent my time dreaming. It felt like being in love, when love is returned. Life could not have been more perfect.

Like anything romanticized, reality strikes too soon. Here I was, living my dream and yet wishing I could be on dry, solid land, far away from seasickness and seasick people.

With all the self-control I could muster, I controlled my gag reflex and tossed a plastic bucket to the woman, muttering my sympathies. I hurried out of the bathroom, past the sweltering engine room, and into the lounge. Thankfully, I had thought to bring my small blanket with me.

More cold sweat beaded on my face. I surveyed the room of miserable sailors. The bodies of staff and volunteers littered benches along the walls and beanbags on the floor, all trying to survive. A few seafarers chatted happily together, completely unaffected. Once more, envy rose within me.

I crawled to an empty spot on a bench, curled up, and willed myself to sleep. My routine soon became: wake up, take seasickness medicine, eat a dry biscuit, drink water, return to sleep, repeat every few hours. During one of my waking moments, a friend emerged from his shift in the engine room. He took one look at my tanned-turned-ashen face and smiled.

"You don't sail so well," he said, playfully tapping my leg with his arm, cheeky grin across his face.

"Please do not make me talk," is all I could gasp. He laughed and threw himself into a beanbag, falling to sleep almost immediately.

Eventually, I awoke to the engine shifting. We had slowed.

The sun streamed in through the lounge windows. People moved about the ship. Life seemed to be returning. I peered out the window for my first glimpse of the remote Papua New Guinea. Tiny figures of children ran across the shoreline, excitedly waving. Dense palms and vegetation spread as far as the eye could see.

We anchored at the mouth of the Bamu River in the Western Province. My seasickness was almost forgotten. Like many rivers in PNG, the Bamu is miles wide but shallow. Shifting sandbanks, rising and falling with the ocean tides, make navigation treacherous. This meant a limited time frame for our ship to get up river. It also meant strategic navigation with a sea-scope for our captain.

The next day was gloomy and rainy. However, it would not deter the curious few who wanted to make their way to shore. Oropai was our first stop. Like so many other villages in PNG, it was small and situated along the banks. In this case, it was on Uapumba Island at the Bamu's broad mouth.

If there is one word I could use to describe my time in the Western Province, I would sum it up with *muddy*. The rainy season in PNG lasts about six months of the year where, essentially, the Western Province becomes shrouded in heavy gray clouds. The rain falls in a slow patter of droplets or in sheets of deluge. The only difference between the wet and dry seasons is that during the dry season the sun comes out after the rain.

Between river rising and falling with ocean tides and the unending rain, the landscape turns muddy.

It was Sunday; the clinics were not starting until the following day. The people of Oropai's curiosity matched ours, so not long after sunrise, dugout canoes pulled up alongside our ship. The sea door was open and we began to see faces peering around the corners. Our ship had about eight Papua New Guinean volunteers who greeted their brothers from Oropai and talked with them. Tok Pisin is the trade language of PNG, but over 800 languages in a nation of seven million makes for some communication difficulties.

Our crew hailed from places like Milne Bay, Central Province, and the Highlands of PNG, all far removed from the Western Province. Their local dialects were not remotely similar to those of the Bamu Region. Also, the Bamu was the poorest region in the poorest province of PNG. Many of the locals were not well-traveled or educated, making them less likely to speak Tok Pisin, let alone English.

After the initial communication was completed, explaining we would be in tomorrow for clinics, the dugout canoes made their way back to shore.

We loaded up in an inflatable dinghy, known as a Zodiac, and jetted across the water to Oropai. The tide was receding, which meant the Zodiac could not get too close to the village. With my backpack full of camera gear, I swung my legs over the side, dropping into calf-deep mud. Unlike sandy shores, the mud here had a soft, claylike quality making it hard to walk or keep balance. Each step created a vacuum beneath my feet. Mud squished between my toes. Shoes were pointless and, had I been wearing any, would have been sucked off my feet.

Each step was slick and I had to concentrate to keep from tumbling over. An amazing world was unfolding before my eyes. Small crabs scurried across the banks in and out of tiny holes in the mud; I hoped I would miss stepping on them. From time to time, coconut shells and other natural debris hidden under the mud surprised us, cutting our feet. The twenty-five yard trek felt like a mile by the time we made it to the slippery ladders propped against the natural shoreline created by high tides.

I climbed up to the village. The people of Oropai grinned ear-to-ear. I was unsure if this was because they were happy to see us or if our clumsy slog through the muddy beach was entertaining. I suspected that it was the latter. In my ignorance, I did not realize how ritualistic a deep mud hike would become over the next few weeks as the high tides rarely cooperated with our schedule.

Our small group greeted and played with the local children, while our leaders met with the village elders, getting an idea of the best places to set up clinics for the following day and their needs. As this was my first encounter with PNG hospitality, their generosity astounded me. Green coconuts, a gift of friendship, appeared from every side.

As the official photographer, I took hundreds of photos. Everything was new and exciting. I was finally here, living my dream. It was muddier than I had anticipated but at least I was not seasick anymore.

One of the things that intrigued me most was the locals' mode of transportation. The jungle terrain was too dense and harsh to travel through, so the rivers became highways. Coastal Papua New Guineans are remarkable seafarers. In handmade dugout canoes with outriggers added, they can navigate rough, swift, flowing waters. Some canoes had sails patched together from many different tarps and scraps of material. It was a sign of ingenuity, skill, and an adept ability to survive: human resilience at its best.

A few days later, I experienced riding in an old dinghy with a patchwork sail on the open water. It was absolutely terrifying. I believed the rough waters would capsize us and take me out to sea. I am an excellent swimmer and I had a life vest, but I felt certain that either drowning or becoming bait for the saltwater crocodiles that inhabited those waters was in my future. Thankfully, the men sailing the vessel were significantly more competent than I had credited them. We arrived at our destination without incident.

As a rock climber, I was captivated by locals nimbly climbing palm trees for coconuts with nothing but small notches cut into the sides of the tree. They effortlessly moved up and down the towering palms. At the top, they called out and dropped the heavy mortars. I was tempted to join them but was pretty confident I would not be able to get down from the top.

Once harvested, they husked the coconut using a sharp stick angled out of the ground. Thrusting the coconut down onto the point, they would twist, ripping off the husk. It took only seconds. With the husk removed, the back of a machete would crack the hard shell with a few skilled hits, exposing the meat for a tasty snack. Green coconuts make refreshing drinks with their tops punctured.

My fascination with the new and exciting would soon be tried by the harsh realities of poverty and purpose. My romantic ideals were about to be reformed. As a well-traveled writer and photographer who grew up in third world nations, I still had much to learn.

Our mission in the Western Province was to provide healthcare, support community development, and improve future opportunities via relationships and education, while meeting PNG's National Health Care plan standard. It was the medical ship's first year in the Bamu Region, which was an important step in the community's development due to their exceptional medical need and isolation.

Deakin University put out a report in 2012 stating: Robert Mugabe's Zimbabwe has the lowest level of human development and is ranked 137, at the very bottom, Professor McGillivray said. The conflict-affected Democratic Republic of Congo is ranked 136. Yet if the resource-rich Western Province was a country, it would be ranked in between Zimbabwe and Congo, and as such among the three very poorest in the world in terms of human development.

Clinics began the next day. Zodiacs carried loads of doctors, nurses, eye care teams, and supplies to the shore. The dentists stayed on the *M/V Pacific Link* in its clinic while patients were transported to and fro (mostly) for tooth extractions.

I went ashore with a team. This time, the Zodiac was able to get closer to the banks. My job was to photograph clinics and gather stories. The previous day, we had met a handful of families; today, hundreds—several from nearby villages—lined up to greet our teams. Customary to coastal homes, the buildings are built upon stilts to prevent flooding when the tides and rains wash over the shores. Front yards become part of the river several times a year, making it difficult to sustain gardens and crops. The primary healthcare clinic was set up in Oropai's largest structure. About five feet above ground, it consisted of a floor, a wall on one side, and a roof of thatched palm leaves. The cross-planked floors groaned beneath the weight of medical supplies, our team, and the lined-up patients.

The team spent the majority of their time giving vital immunizations, prenatal care, and cleaning wounds. Our research showed that these are the most important short-term needs; one in seven women in remote PNG die in childbirth and one in thirteen children die under the age of five. Wound care was another immediate need; it helped to stave off infection due to tropical conditions and lack of sanitation. A small cut could threaten limb and life if left untreated.

The optical team spent time testing eyes and finding spectacles for patients who had not seen clearly for years. Better eyesight improved daily living, the ability to farm, hunt, fish, and navigate the waters. While the primary healthcare clinic consisted of screaming children in fear of immunizations, the optometry clinic was full of happy people who celebrated being able to see again. Both clinics were incredibly busy. In addition to our clinics, I also witnessed our midwives teaching local women about birth and pre- and post-natal care.

One of the risks of working in the village was the stability of the building from which we operated. In Oropai, as more and more people filtered through, the floor on the far side of the clinic gave a frightful crack. I looked over in time to see an entire section of people and medical instruments drop from sight with screams. The quick-thinking nurses saved the immunizations before they could tumble over the edge. As I hurried to help, people had already picked themselves up from the mud. Minutes later, the planks were replaced and medical care resumed as if nothing happened.

We wrapped up our first day without much more incident.

Routine soon set in as we traveled to a new village each day. We trudged through knee-deep mud in Sisiami 2, Piripuri, Mirowu, Bamio, and Emeti to name a few. In our third village, Mirowu, came one of my biggest wake up calls to the plight of this region.

Daru was the closest hospital, a few days travel in open waters in a dinghy, possibly less if a person had an outboard motor and petrol, which most didn't. As a result, many women gave birth in their villages. That morning, as clinics started, we were alerted to a woman experiencing labor pains on the verge of childbirth. The midwife checked her and was happy to see that the baby looked healthy and in good position.

It was an especially rainy morning. I had hesitated to even break out my camera for fear it would get too wet.

Due to a stigma around birth and a general lack of knowledge, many women in this region are forced to give birth outdoors, regardless of weather conditions. For Bokoro, this was no exception. That day, she gave birth to her second child, a girl, under a makeshift shelter while sitting on a wood sheet in ankle deep mud. Blood mixed with water and mud, as the final stages of the birthing process took place. Once alerted, our team arrived in time to assist her delivery.

After cleaning the baby and wrapping mother and child in donated blankets, the team insisted that Bokoro and the baby be allowed back in her home where a warm fire could be built. Often, women remain outside until the postpartum bleeding subsides, making them significantly more susceptible to illness and death. A community healthcare worker informed us that in many villages in this region they believe men will get sick [with coughing and shortness of breath] if they see blood related to birth.

I followed the midwife back to Bokoro's home later that day for an interview as immunizations and a check-up were administered. Little did I know how involved I would become in the process. The midwife slipped and fell into a muddy creek on our way. Thankfully the immunizations had been safely placed inside a rubber glove and were protected during the fall. She, however, was nowhere near clean enough to administer the injections. We were too far from the clinic to turn back. It fell on me, the media. I slathered on hand sanitizer and let her skilled hands guide mine through immunizing the newborn. I held the needle; she held my hand. Terror gripped me as the baby's cry rose with the first poke, but I knew the shot could preserve her little life in the long run.

I began to realize that the Land of the Unexpected truly lived up to its name.

IN THE VALLEY

In our attempts to make a lasting impact, we hoped Boroko's labor would help more than one woman and child. Through educating the people of the village, we started breaking down the superstitions surrounding childbirth with the hope that future mothers would be able to give birth in better conditions. My experience led me to believe that although the people have a mother's best interest at heart, they do not understand the value of sanitation during childbirth. One of our primary goals was to educate the Bamu Region's people in order to bring them towards a healthier quality of life.

As the weeks wore on, the mud and precipitation lost all appeal. I was tired of being wet and slipping from village to village, clinic to clinic. I was grateful at the end of each day for a hot shower back on the *M/V Pacific Link* and clean attire. All the while, I recognized that the villagers did not have this luxury.

I remember lying in my bunk at night, wrestling with the injustice of poverty. Despite my knowledgeable worldview, I had never experienced anything like the Western Province. What amazed me was the incredible resilience of the people. Every day, they rise and fight nature and odds to survive. Where I am from, we complain if we wait an hour at the doctor's; these villagers paddle the open sea for days to see a doctor. I met blind people who journeyed across a province for eye surgery. When all the odds appear against them, remote Papua New Guineans relentlessly believe it could get better.

I learned in deeper ways it was possible to have joy despite lacking every material possession. I learned that insurmountable obstacles seemed to propel some people to embrace life. I learned that hope can be sustained in any circumstance.

What broke my heart, however, was not the physical poverty, but the spiritual despondency. What can you do when people give up on life? How can you blame them? Much like falling in love, I had thrilling moments with butterflies and gloried in the newness of it, but I also faced the pain of my ideals being confronted while tough life questions were presented.

I found a small hidey-hole on the ship where I tucked myself away to have a good cry and grapple with it all. I watched the brown river waves lap up against the side of the ship, pondering how many crocodiles lived below the surface.

My love for PNG came to its shadowed valley in a village called Bamio. It had been over a week since I had seen the sun when we arrived at Bamio. The area felt shrouded in thick clouds. The tide was at its lowest. This meant an extra-long trek through the mud.

I almost fell off a few slick logs that bridged the swamp drains and was tired of the locals laughing at my faltering steps and grabbing my elbows to propel me along. I was exhausted and had cuts on my feet, I was wet, I was muddy, and I did not want to be in Bamio. The novelty had gone. I could no longer see the beauty in their faces nor hear the happiness in their laughter. I saw old, ripped clothing on gaunt bodies. I saw hopelessness. This was one of the poorest regions in the poorest province. Its staggering statistics made one wonder how anyone could overcome the mounting negative odds against them. Food was scarce. Medical care and clean water, even more so.

We went to follow up on baby Umi, whom our crew had discovered on their previous outreach to this village. She was 1.7 kilograms, or about three and a half pounds, at two months old because her mother travelled long distances to work in the fields. While she harvested sago, Umi was left at home with her siblings. Without enough material to tie the baby to herself, her mother would be gone for at least eight hours a day while the baby was left unfed. In a place where muddy jungle treks or canoe rides were the transportation, a mother had to carry her child somehow. Baby-wearing via bilum or sling is a common practice in PNG, however, this village lacked enough resources to even make those.

After education and the help of nurses on the last visit, we hoped Umi was still alive and progressing. We found her family but immediately heard sad news. The father had lost his battle with tuberculosis the previous week.

Much to our delight, however, Umi was alive and had gained half a kilo. She was still dangerously underweight, but we saw hope. Unfortunately, the loss of the father had left the mother despondent. Barely lifting her eyes, the frail woman mourned deeply. Her toddler son clung to her side as she cradled Umi in her lap. Our joy over the baby's progress seemed to fall on deaf ears.

How do you share hope with people who have lost their loved ones to preventable disease? How do you encourage someone when they are barely surviving? Her sad eyes haunted me. My friend, Adriel, is a mother and wife. With an understanding sympathy, she gently comforted the woman, offering solace as a peer who understood the significance of this loss. Her own heart broke in a way that would inspire her to fight for change in maternal health.

DEFINING MY PURPOSE

Later that day, I took photos in the clinic as people filtered through it. My awakening drew near. A sick little boy was about to teach me my purpose.

A mother brought in her three-year-old son who had lost all use of the left side of his body. He was clearly on the verge of death. As I looked into the face of the little boy, I saw the end stages of tuberculosis consuming his tiny body.

I heard one of the Australian nurses gasp. She looked at me, asking, "What happened to that child?"

I burst into tears and fled to a back room of the clinic. Sitting among medical supplies, tears spilled down my face. The little boy's mother barely registered emotion. She had brought her son into the clinic knowing there was likely no hope for him. I could not begin to comprehend what holding a dying child was like.

Adriel and I interviewed mothers in Bamio. Almost all of them had lost at least one child. One woman threw her hands up in despair, crying. All three of her children had perished. They were not statistics; they were faces, people I sat with, cried with, prayed for, and whose hands I held.

There was nothing romantic about this field work. There was no grand ideal emerging through my job. The giddiness of romanticized daydreams had faded, but love remained. In the hard moments, I fell more in love with the people and PNG. There were times I felt helpless to do anything about the plight of the poor and needy. At one point, I looked upon the medical staff with envy. They made a visible and immediate impact on hundreds of people daily while all I did was take photographs and write.

Sitting on the ship at the end of the day, Adriel and I talked about Bamio. Her two beautiful little boys played around us. Emotion washed over me as I told her about Wesley, the little boy dying from TB. I could see the pain in her eyes as well. Pausing with reflection she looked at me and responded, "Write about it. Tell their story."

I picked up Adriel's youngest, Judah, cuddling him as I looked at his healthy little face. Tears brimmed in my eyes as I thought about how much I wanted the children in PNG to be as healthy and happy as he was. Judah had two healthy parents who loved him, he had a full belly, he had the freedom to play and learn, he had access to good medical care, he was vaccinated against so many of the life-threatening diseases the children of Papua New Guinea would perish from.

Sitting in my on-ship hiding place, watching the sunset across the waters, the realization washed over me. I could tell their stories. I could keep their memories alive in the hopes that one day people would care enough to bring more lasting community development to PNG and its remote provinces. One day, through raising awareness, the chains of poverty binding them may be just a memory.

I could tell the world. They are people, like you and me. Poverty does not diminish their value. They have hopes, desires, and dreams. They are resilient.

My life verse came back to mind, Proverbs 31:8-9: "Open your mouth for the mute, for the rights of all who are destitute. Open your mouth, judge righteously, defend the rights of the poor and needy."

The story does not end there. A year later, we followed up and found that baby Umi was alive and "fatter," according to the locals. There is hope.

Not only did Adriel inspire me, she started "Love a Mama Community." Her initiatives include: **Bloggers for Birth Kits:** providing clean birth kits for women in remote, underdeveloped areas; **Project Baby Bilum:** getting ring slings to mamas who otherwise have to leave their newborns behind while they gather food for their families; **The Sunshine Project:** solar suitcases used for emergency obstetrics, midwifery, and other medical work when power is not available; and she supports an initiative called **Days for Girls:** sanitary options for girls and women in the developing world.

I learned we do not need to reinvent the wheel or seek out someone else's divinely-inspired gift to change the world. We need to be exactly who we are to make a positive impact on people and places. Medicine is not my calling. I learned I need to be myself, seasick, muddy, artsy, wordy, little me.

TELLING THE KAPUNA LEGACY

I returned to Australia more passionate than ever about healthcare in remote regions. Seasons came and went as I transitioned into other jobs on staff, growing and learning. As I helped remodel our buildings, my days consisted of painting, painting, and more painting. It was a nice transition from the busier work I had been doing but with paint spattered legs and aching arms, I acknowledged, I did not want to be here forever. I had just turned 30 and was reflecting on life.

A theme that has emerged throughout my life was growing beyond just journalism. I had always dreamed of writing a book but was never fully inspired by a topic, until now.

What if I put together an accumulation of stories from Papua New Guinea? I could possibly do even more traveling throughout the nation, continuing to connect. Over the next few weeks, I could not shake the idea. I knew I needed to filter my ideas through a leader with experience.

Adriel and her husband, Ryan, immediately came to mind. I contacted her; we sat down one afternoon to talk. Her enthusiasm was overwhelming. She is also a writer. As we talked, she shared ideas and vision. I was encouraged. However, they did not believe it would be possible to tackle such a project while on staff with the organization. There were too many roles to fill. Taking time out of work to write a book might be asking too much.

I knew what I needed to do. The question was: where, when, and how?

With the orange glow of campfire warming our faces, Beth Lewis shared a piece of her history with me. Sitting on a log in the chilly mountain air of North Queensland, Australia, this young British doctor poured out her love for Papua New Guinea. I was captivated. She shared bits of her upbringing, traveling to China, her family's Christmas adventures including cold outdoor picnics, her anthropologist father, her life as a medical student living on next to nothing, her residency work in a remote Western Province hospital in Papua New Guinea, and her plans to move to Kapuna, Gulf Province to work as a doctor.

Months later, when she had settled in to Kapuna, updates from her life as a bush doctor came pouring in. She shared victories mingled with tragedies and frustrations: a life saved, a life lost, crazy illnesses and injuries, alongside hilarious mishaps. It was July 2013. I had just had the conversation with Adriel about writing my book when I sensed I should talk to Beth. While I did not know her well at the time, she had shared the long hours of her job and the weight of just losing a patient. Sending her a private message, I asked her if we could chat.

A few nights later, with the evening encroaching, I swung in my hammock getting ready to Skype Dr. Beth. Through pouring out her first few months as a doctor in Kapuna, one thing was clear: Dr. Beth was in love with Papua New Guinea and her job. Through the struggles and triumphs, I could not help but be touched by her gratitude for her work and each new day. It struck me how appreciative she was for the opportunity to build relationships with her patients, not just see them once and send them to outpatient. She got to know their names and their families, she fought for them, and she followed up on them. She shared that back in England she could patch people up, but she would never be allowed to pray for them. Here in the bush, she could share her faith as well as her skill.

She recognized that her knowledge was continuously being stretched. There was a never ending evolution of skills in Kapuna Hospital. If a surgery was needed, the doctors did the surgery; if treatment for a rare illness was needed, they did their best to treat it; if a baby was to be born, they delivered it. Each day, each problem allowed for flexibility and a vast expanse of learning.

She unveiled another story of this little hospital on the banks of a river, with an 88-year-old doctor who had been there since the 1950s. She still did rounds. It was a story of resiliency and incredible faithfulness. As our conversation neared its end, a thought bubbled to the surface.

"Beth?" I eagerly broke out, "How do you think they would feel if I came out and wrote a book about Kapuna?"

She responded enthusiastically. At the time, I sensed she did not realize how serious I was about this. I am not sure I knew how seriously I was about this. All I knew is this was the story I was supposed to tell about PNG. This is where I would start. I had no idea about the when, but I now knew the where.

Amazingly enough, a few months later, the pieces fell into place.

THE JOURNAL ENTRY

In the midst of writing this book, I went back and found this gem in my journal. A common character trait in me is the ability to find unfavorable adventure and unwitting twists to my life stories. Naturally, the journey to Kapuna Hospital began this way for me.

I arrived in Papua New Guinea yesterday. Despite what was supposed to be very exciting, I am very unimpressed with that moment in life.

It had started as any other chaotic day of leaving one's old life behind and pressing on into the new. No matter how far in advance I start packing, I never seem to be ready when the time comes to leave. So many last minute things!

A 5 a.m. alarm pulled me groggily into reality as I slid off my top bunk for the last time, hit the ground too hard because I always underestimate the distance to the ground, and tip-toed around to not wake up my roommate while I finished packing. I plucked my clean clothing that had been drying off the backs of chairs (I did not want to risk leaving them on the line if it might rain), rolled them up, and stuffed them into my tightly expanding pack. Just one more inch to fill!

Shoving and grunting, I cinched it closed only to remember one more thing.

Before I leave on trips I have check lists and back-up check lists. I checked and rechecked that I packed all of the important things. For the 75th time I made sure my passport was in my bag; that I actually had exchanged my money and it wasn't a dream; and, I did remember to save all of the important phone numbers in three different locations in three different bags.

You laugh, but I'm always the one prepared!

The one thing I did not throw in my carry-on, however, was my migraine pills.

"Seriously, what are the odds I'd get one today?" I thought.

Next time, they will be riding in my carry-on. That was a foolish moment. But, sure, I have hand sanitizer that smells like cranberries!

My friend, Melissa, drove me to the airport. I was not too emotional about leaving. I never am. My emotions will hit me at a later, completely inappropriate time. I will cry uncontrollably over something insignificant because it will be then in that moment the weight of saying "goodbye" and moving to the bush of Papua New Guinea will finally hit me.

However, when Melissa offered to pray for me, the tears streamed down my face. She is a sweet little sister to me. We had been on our journey with Youth With A Mission from the very beginning of our Discipleship Training School (DTS) until now. I truly love Australia and the people in my life there.

We hugged and I left to check in for my flight.

Leaving Townsville was uneventful. The flight to Cairns is less than an hour. It was smooth. I gazed out the window at the Great Barrier Reef and fluffy white clouds most of the way. A small headache had started but I figured I was just tired.

By the time I got off the plane and lugged my carry-ons—I've never learned to pack light—to the International Terminal, the air had changed and rain started to pour down. My headache was a lot worse.

I stopped in the bathroom before going through Customs and Security. As I bent over the room started to spin and full blown migraine cracked across my brain.

I dug through my bag looking for medicine of any kind. Aspirin. That will do! I popped the pills as quickly as I could into my mouth, praying I had time before I could not even stand up any more. I gagged on the water I went to wash it down with. Not a good sign.

As I stood at the desk of the Immigrations officer looking at my passport, I had to lean on the counter to hold myself up. I started to sweat profusely. I felt too sick to even talk. I thought they might pull me aside because I looked suspicious, sweating and not making eye contact.

The only thing my brain could focus on was, "Don't throw up, don't throw up, oh God help me, I am going to throw up."

I dropped my carry-ons into the trays and prepared for the items to go through security. I passed through the metal detector, gagged, and sprinted to the closest bin.

I emptied the contents of my stomach into the rubbish bin.

Thankfully, Australian airport security personal tend to be very friendly. A concerned woman brought me some paper towels and helped me sit down. She had set aside all of my stuff. I thought I was the past the worst. Surely, it could not get worse than this?

Migraines come in waves. It eased for a bit so I took my things and headed for my gate. By the time I sat down, I was fighting nausea again. I had two hours. All I could do was close my eyes. I slept, or rather, passed out: head tilted back and mouth wide open.

Just for the record, I do not normally sleep well anywhere, let alone airports. A sure sign I am sick is if I can doze in odd places.

I boarded the plane and my headache was far from gone. I immediately fell asleep on the flight, only to wake from time to time and think, "Please don't throw up." Or, "My head is going to explode."

They handed out food.

People say pregnant ladies have the noses of a bloodhound, but I'm pretty sure migraines give me super-human senses.

If this is what food smells like to pregnant ladies, then my heart goes out to them. Ham sandwiches have never smelled stronger or more disgusting than on that flight. I could smell each grain of wheat in the bread. It was like the ham had been slaughtered and baked in front of me. I declined all food and beverage except water.

As fearful as I usually am of flying, I don't think I would have minded if both engines had cut and we plummeted into the ocean. Anything was better than this headache. We finally landed in Port Moresby but my head was at full explosive state.

We started to deplane and I was in no hurry. A handsome, tattooed, Kiwi bodyguard helped me get my bags and started a friendly banter with me. I tried to smile and be gracious but I mostly thought, "I hope I don't vomit on the guy!"

I honestly felt too weak to talk and mostly smiled back at him, wishing inside I could just sit down and die. Then, we arrived at the visa line. Why did every noise in that place have to sound so much louder? Why was every fluorescent light burning a hole in my brain? Why was this guy still talking to me?

Why do men insist on flirting with me when I am at my worst? I was pale, sweaty, in my travel clothes, and I had just been sick at the last airport; not exactly eye-catching material here. Vulnerable? Yes. Attractive? No.

We made it through the first visa line. The man ahead of me got into an argument with the woman at the window.

Apparently she tried to charge him twice. He looked to me for sympathy, but I just wanted him to pay and move on. Then, there was the second visa line. Strength was leaving my body. I seriously considered sitting down in the middle of the line. The cool tile looked appealing. My other thought was to ask strong-handsome-Kiwi-man to carry me the rest of the way. I had no qualms with dangling over his shoulder at this point. I could not focus on anything.

"How long are you here for?"

I looked up to see the visa employee looking at me. I was next in line. I handed over my passport and smiled. The visa man asked me more questions, I could not focus. I wanted to die.

Stamp!

Passport handed back to me. My luggage was pulled off the conveyer belt and sitting on the ground. I grabbed a cart, mostly to prop myself up when I walked. I loaded my bags and fought off nausea. Almost there!

I was stopped at Customs, handed over my papers, asked a few questions. I blabbed something about the YWAM Medical Ship and how I'd been here before to work with them. At those words, the man smiled, said he liked YWAM, and waved me through.

I met up with my friend's parents who were waiting to pick me up. I immediately told them how I felt and we walked to the car.

Once in the car, I knew I'd be sick again. Less than five minutes into the drive, I asked them to pull over.

"Welcome to PNG," I thought as I threw up on a sidewalk along the roadway. I was weak and trembling, almost completely oblivious to the boring eyes of curious bystanders.

They got me to their house, turned on the air-con in my room, and shut the door. Other than one more round of throwing up in a bowl, I covered my eyes with my arm and slept for the next five hours. Even though I have not lived at home for over twelve years, in these moments I really want my mom or dad to be there with me.

While I had many ups-and-downs in preparing to come to PNG, the biggest thing for me was the juggling of the ever changing internal flights. Getting to Kapuna is not an easy task. It requires random flights and boat rides, all coordinated with the safety of the river tides.

I love how God knows the details long before we do. I was supposed to fly to Kapuna today, but due to a series of unfortunate miscommunications, my flight was pushed back. I was so weak and tired today; I cannot even imagine having another flight and boat ride in the heat. I am so grateful I had a few days of rest before continuing my journey.

Maybe God knew I'd have a headache. I love how His timing just always seems to work out better than our own plans.

Go figure, after all of my jokes about my weak stomach and how I've thrown up all over the world, this would be the way I start my new life!

THE HISTORY OF PNG AND KAPUNA

There I was in the copilot's seat of a bush plane, overlooking the veined rivers of Papua New Guinea. With Baimuru station lingering in the distance, our plane slowly descended. We circled the sawmill and the town, as people came running from every direction down below. After landing on the grass airstrip at Baimuru, I was greeted by my friend, Gerald, and soon-to-be friend, Annaleigh, both volunteers at Kapuna Hospital. Walking through swampy grasses, we lugged my bags to Kapuna's aluminum canoe. Sitting atop lumber for the school they were building, we made our journey to Kapuna Hospital.

Traveling up the broad Wame River, a tributary of the Purari River in the Gulf Province of Papua New Guinea, there was a consistent monotony of dense palms and mangroves. Finally the landscape broke at Ara'ava. It was a long village built close to the shores. Muddy banks were lined for a mile or two with homes built up on stilts.

From time to time, drop toilets hovered in rows along the banks. Some were leaning precariously to one side. Canoes were tied to posts all along the shores. As anyone passed, they would be sure to have men, women, and children stop to wave, especially if they were outsiders. Dogs, chickens, a cassowary, and sometimes pigs could also be spotted throughout the village.

After Ara'ava we could see breaks in the bush where banana trees and gardens were planted near the shores. An opening in the banana trees showed a sago station with three stands for beating sago, a local food staple.

Unseen by a person in the boat, a small worn path ran along the river and its gardens up to Kapuna. Many people walked daily back and forth over that same path to take food to the markets, visit family at the hospital, or work in their gardens. They were the closest, most available neighbors to Kapuna Hospital, only a 20-30 minute walk away. The rainy season rendered the pathway navigable by only the most sure-footed people.

Kapuna was much harder to spot due to the surrounding swamp lands. It sat significantly further back from the river. It was easier to identify in the evenings due to the glow of light from generators but a person had to be looking to find it. Tall grass and purple hyacinth extended in front of it.

The long jetty was the indicator for truly arriving at Kapuna. It stretched over the swamp land, out to the river where boats could tie up or follow the narrow inlet, depending on the height of the tides. The long jetty waters meandered past the docking point and into narrow swamp drains wrapping through Kapuna.

Most of the canoes and dinghies made it in to tie up in rows near the hospital. Some volunteers referred to it as our "car park." Here the majority of traffic from this area of the Gulf Province converged. On a daily basis, families would be loading and unloading bedding, clothes, and food for a stay at the hospital. Some traveled days via canoe from their villages.

Immediately, the faded green paint of multiple large buildings greeted us, along with the red rusting corrugated iron roofs. Long covered and raised walkways connected the hospital wards. People rested along the benches throughout the walkways. A cool breeze seemed to flow through bringing relief from the tropical heat. Doctors and nurses in their white uniforms, interns, and community healthcare students in their green uniforms floated from ward to ward, talking to patients, filling prescriptions, and stopping to greet people along the way.

Kapuna physically may consist of faded buildings, but the spirit it exudes is anything but faded or ordinary. It is one incredible place with an even more extraordinary history.

Sixty years earlier, the swampy jungle would have ruled the Kapuna area.

Papua New Guinea is known as one of the last frontiers of the world. With over 800 people groups and as many languages, accompanied by a harsh tropical mountainous landscape, there is still much exploration and understanding of cultures left to do. Due to the tribal isolation, the written history of Melanesia only extends back to the time of colonization.

Archeological evidence, however, suggests the ancestors of modern PNG peoples were among some of the earliest farmers.

While the Dutch ruled the western half of the island of New Guinea, the Germans settled the northern regions of the eastern half, and the British settled the southern portion. The Highlands were divided by these two nations, but remained mostly untouched due to the rugged terrain and inaccessibility. Many tribes in the Highlands stayed completely unaware of lines drawn on imperial maps.

The areas closer to the shores, however, were more affected by colonization as explorers made their way inland. Imagine the fear when the unknown white-skins penetrated the culture, looking very much like spirits and ghosts. British history records the reactions of the locals as being many times hostile, but fails to record the thoughts and terror that the locals associated with having their entire world turned upside down.

The "white-skins" also held the unfair advantage of modern tools of war versus stone axes, spears, and bows and arrows. The natives' knowledge of the rivers, dense jungle, and threatening wildlife is in part what preserved them. While the Europeans had modern technology, the locals were much better equipped to survive the many native perils PNG territory threatened.

Soon after World War I, the German and British rules of the eastern half of New Guinea were handed over to Australia, a new nation at the time.

Once again, in many parts of Papua New Guinea, the people of the nation were neither affected by nor informed of the colonial lines being moved again. Those who had encountered the white-skins were met with pretty much the same experience regardless of whether it was with British, German, or Australian.

One huge effect of globalization and contact with the outside world was the development of Tok Pisin, also known as New Guinea Pidgin. It is one of the most common, widely used languages in Papua New Guinea today: a trade language.

Another effect of contact with the outside world was the arrival of missionaries. In many ways, they shaped much of PNG. Books like Kira Salak's *Four Corners* depict Christian missionaries in Papua New Guinea in less than glowing accounts. Their selfishness and desire to change the culture of

PNG left a negative impact on her, and understandably so. However, those she encountered were only a small fraction of the people and organizations spread throughout the Land of the Unexpected. In fairness, like any other occupation or lifestyle, despite those negatively depicted, there are many who handle adversity and change with grace, those who have more cultural awareness than others, those who are in PNG for the right reasons, and those who do not burn out as quickly as some. My research brought up a swinging pendulum of opinions and information on this topic.

Research in his graduate dissertation by sociologist, Robert Woodberry, states,

> Areas where Protestant missionaries had a significant presence in the past are on average more economically developed today, with comparatively better health, lower infant mortality, lower corruption, greater literacy, higher educational attainment (especially for women), and more robust membership in nongovernmental associations.

His research was not specifically done on the nation of Papua New Guinea, but covered missionary reaches throughout the world.

Robert Petterson, a New Zealand native who has lived in Papua New Guinea on and off since the 1980s shared his extensive knowledge on the topic. He said, "From our remote viewpoint, colonization and missionaries seem connected because they appear to happen simultaneously, but in fact they were independent movements and should not be linked too closely. Colonies did not necessarily settle with the arrival of European powers. Missionaries sometimes preceded, sometimes followed on from the arrival of administrators of European powers, and sometimes called on help from those powers to protect indigenous peoples from exploitation by ruthless opportunists (e.g., in New Zealand). They had different goals too. Missionaries promoted literacy in local languages from the late 1800s, but the Australian administration, when it at last took an interest in education in the 1950s, promoted and funded education in English only. Many early missionaries to PNG were, in fact, Pacific Islanders. Also, colonization often implies significant settlements of Europeans, as happened in Australia and New Zealand but not in PNG. In PNG it was an exploitative type of small-scale colonization (e.g., beche-de-mer trading and coconut plantations!) governed by an overseas-based administration. New Zealand, on the other hand, underwent a massive European land-grab with clearance of forests and conversion to sheep and dairy. Missionaries tried very hard to defend Maori rights, but eventually lost, resulting in the 1860 land wars. This sort of thing did not happen in PNG. The land is still owned by the indigenous population, and they rule themselves." He continued, "The biggest negative effects on modern culture here come from corruption, foreign investment, AIDS, violence, drugs—hardly from missionaries. It is very true that both missionaries *and* government administration had effects on culture, but whether positive or negative depends on your values: sorcery vs medicine, initiation vs education, sickness vs health, tribal fighting, fear and cannibalism vs peace, communication and cooperation, traditional art and song forms vs imported global art and music. I say 'why not retain the old as well as take in the popular new?' It can be hard to stem the tide of desired change. Many of our older PNG friends shake their heads in horror of how things were when they were children, and are so grateful for the arrival of the gospel of peace to come and save their tribe, allowing them to live and travel in freedom and without fear today."

The biggest loss of traditional culture follows on from pacification by the administration and subsequent opening up of opportunities to travel and see how other people live.

Gulf Province people took these opportunities with great interest. A famous local example is Tommy Kabo, who escaped to Australia during the Japanese invasion. He observed the Australian way of life and commerce, and returned to the Gulf after the war and persuaded his people to burn down all the longhouses and make villages in better places where they could set up commercial trading operations. (He was a Bahai, not a Christian.)

The government anthropologist documenting the famous and complex Orokolo celebrations noted that regrettably they would soon inevitably be lost because of contact with the outside world and opportunities for travel and commerce.

A couple of months ago I heard an old man blame the loss of the Motu language on the Christian religion. This is a misconception.

Christian missionaries devised an alphabet and translated the Bible into the Motu language, and used it as a trade language and for pastor training. It was not suppressed at all. What has contributed to the loss of Motu was the flood of settlers from other regions speaking Tok Pisin as they came into Motu speaking areas. This has nothing to do with Christianity, government, or whatever. It is more an effect of urban drift or globalization."

Tales of cannibalized white-skins have filtered out to the rest of the world through the years. Some of these stories were confirmed by tribes in the highlands to a group of my friends trekking through in 2011. My friends met an elder of one tribe who informed them that the last missionaries in the area, about fifty years earlier, were killed and eaten by him and his fellow clan members. He asked for forgiveness for his lack of understanding of why the white-skin was there.

In complete contrast to the events of cannibalism, a PNG dentist friend of mine, Vasiti Kep, shared her family's history with me. When missionaries infiltrated the Mendi area of the Southern Highlands, her family was one of the first to welcome them. Her family helped settle the missionaries into a home in the area; soon after, her family converted to Christianity. They were among the first to build the local church, and donated the land for it.

Vasiti's maternal grandmother was the translator for the Baptist missionaries; she travelled all over Papua New Guinea and even to Australia working alongside them.

One of the many foreign mission organizations to start work in Papua New Guinea was the London Missionary Society (LMS). It was formed in 1795 as a non-denominational mission to reach Africa and the South Pacific. Their work in PNG was validated by sending over 300 Samoans as missionaries to Papua in 1844. The effects of Samoan culture can still be found throughout PNG.

Kapuna Hospital was formed out of LMS's work, propelled by an anonymous donation in 1949. The scope of the area reached by LMS stretched along the southern coast of PNG, from Daru, Western Province to Samarai, Milne Bay Province.

At the time, they believed the best use for the money was to promote healthcare in one of the neediest areas, the Purari River Delta in the Gulf Province.

Carved out of the dense bush on the Wame River, it was strategically placed for two reasons: it was in a deeper river region, making navigation of bigger vessels easier, and a sawmill across the river could provide the timber for building the hospital.

Soon after the donation, a New Zealand builder led a team of local builders from the Kikori area to erect the hospital buildings. Little did anyone know at the time that there would be an invisible link tying New Zealand to this remote location.

Once the first buildings were completed, Dr. Neville Anderson and his wife, Pat, of Australia made Kapuna Hospital their home. They were the only doctors available to care for tens of thousands of villagers in the area. The remoteness of the area combined with the extreme cultural differences took their toll on the doctor's wife.

Providentially, the hospital, however, was about to receive two doctors who would change the entire face of healthcare and community in the Purari Delta region: the Calverts from New Zealand. This humble family, guided by their deeply rooted faith in God, would create a legacy that spanned generations and does not look like it will end anytime soon.

THE CALVERTS

Petite, blond-hair, blue-eyed Linnie Bryant Tombleson had promised God she would become a missionary. This New Zealand sheep farm girl was oblivious as to how God would employ her promise. In an emotional reaction to a missionary woman who spoke at her Christian college, Lin threw up the prayer and did not think much else of it for years. Raised in a traditional Christian family, she was aware of God's calling, but never suspected how far her faith would be stretched.

It was the early 1940s and she was going to pursue medicine.

Young Peter Calvert made history in his cub pack by fainting at the mere mention of blood. Thinking he had no future as a doctor, he began to pursue law when World War II put a pause on his education. He went to England to serve as a navigator in the Royal Air Force. Returning to New Zealand a different man, he realized he had lost his passion for law but had an interest in medicine after all.

Despite the three year difference in school, the pleasant male medical student caught Lin's eye. Apparently, her beautiful face did not go unnoticed by him either.

Dr. Lin wrote, "Just a few days after he graduated we were married and soon we began to look around for our life's work.

A letter from the London Missionary Society arrived just as we were leaving one day to go to see a film. I have forgotten the film but will never forget the letter which we read in the interval. 'Kapuna is situated in the low-lying swampy delta country of Papua. There would be plenty of opportunity for your wife to share in the medical work. There has been no doctor there for a year. A nursing sister is taking care of the hospital until we can find one.' That sounded fine, just what we wanted, but there was just one small problem—we were not quite sure where Papua was! After the film we went to the public library and found a map."

After spending a year in Sydney pursuing post-graduate qualifications in tropical medicine, Dr. Peter and Dr. Lin Calvert traveled for six weeks, via ship, to Papua New Guinea with their young daughter, Valerie, and new baby boy, Edward (Ted).

At the time, the Australian-ruled government of Papua New Guinea encouraged pioneering work by missionaries, and personally welcomed them. Although the Calverts were coming as medical professionals, their overarching goal was to love people and share the Gospel of Jesus Christ with those around them. Their lives, their medical care, and building the local church were to be witness of the faith inside of them.

Almost immediately after their ship docked in Port Moresby in 1954, they were asked to be ready in professional dress to meet the Governor General—representative for the King or Queen of England in Papua New Guinea.

After a short stay in Port Moresby, the Calverts made their way to Kapuna in the Gulf Province. How could they know the extent to which this bush hospital would truly become home?

The remoteness of Kapuna was about to offer Dr. Peter and Dr. Lin a set of challenges not many could endure. If you were to go to Kapuna Hospital today, you would find generators to run power for a few hours a day or for emergency needs at the hospital, a satellite dish to use internet (that works most of the time), narrow cement sidewalks to keep your feet out of the mud, an aluminum canoe with an outboard motor to get around, and a number of staff homes that mix PNG design with a few Western amenities like indoor plumbing.

Back in 1954, however, the rainy season rendered Kapuna muddy for at least six months. Kerosene lamps or wood fires were all that lit the area at night. Thankfully, there was a kerosene refrigerator to keep vaccines cool.

The only form of communication with the outside world was the boats that came through every few months, bringing mail and supplies. Travel occurred by dugout paddle canoe or by "Martha," a slow chug-chug launch.

There were also very few schools, no English spoken, and as Dr. Lin told me, "This was back when people did not wear clothes, or at least not much more than grass skirts." It was a far stretch from the cultural norms of the south island of New Zealand.

When it was not raining, the grass grew at alarming rates. To avoid the surprise of snakes, especially death adders, the staff would mow with serif, which are sharpened strips of metal. To this day, the same dexterous hands of Dr. Lin that performed countless surgeries are out in the gardens and hospital grounds, skillfully destroying weeds with machete and serif.

Peter, Lin, Valerie, and Ted quickly settled in and made Kapuna home.

The hospital consisted of four thatch-roofed buildings connected by the veranda.

The family expanded as Alan and Colin were later born. Drs. Peter and Lin spent their time working in the hospital, as well as educating and raising four children. The Calverts' work was pioneering to say the least. It was a time of hysterical mishaps mixed with intense moments of spiritual and physical breakthrough.

Dr. Peter was developing solutions to improve the surrounding area medically. He started a radio "medical sked," giving advice to mission stations all over the nation. This service became quickly and hugely popular, although not easy for Dr. Peter. Advice had to suit the conditions, the medicines available, and the competence of those at the other end of the SW (short wave) radio. This was made more difficult through the hiss and crackle of static. The whole family soon learned the radio alphabet.

Peter also spent his time setting up fifteen aid posts throughout the area. He even wrote a manual for training the aid workers.

This program developed into his and Lin's training school at Kapuna. The 51st graduation for the community healthcare workers (CHW) commenced in the front lawn of the hospital in February 2014. It was strong evidence for the lasting impact of the work started so many years ago.

Peter also expanded the work of the village health patrols that went out to villages in the surrounding area. He worked hard and achieved immunization coverage that is said to have rivaled modernized Western countries. Initially, all of his travel was done via canoe, but Mission Aviation Fellowship (MAF) later joined in the efforts advancing and expanding the work with their float plane. MAF uses aviation and technology to reach isolated areas of the world. Their planes and pilots are strategically placed in some of the hardest to reach places on the globe, so they can serve the people through flying in humanitarian workers, aide, missionaries, doctors, etc...

The bush offered an array of surgical challenges. One time, when Dr. Peter was performing a surgery with no electricity, he had new nurses there to assist and hold the torches for him. As the surgery proceeded, whether it was due to their newness or the heat, the nurses fainted. Only one remained to the end, giving him light to see and assistance as needed.

GROWING UP IN PNG

While Dr. Peter and Dr. Lin were busy with the hospital and multiple community development projects, their four children were reveling in the jungle life. The Calverts were well assimilated to the PNG way of life. In fact, other than their bright blue eyes and fair skin, the four Calvert children had a relatively typical Land of the Unexpected upbringing.

Their world included machete skills, understanding and respecting the swamp wildlife, many near-drowning experiences, and learning to navigate a boat before a car. This also led to a myriad of close-calls and hilarious mishaps.

Ted shared a lot of his childhood memories and started by saying, "When I read *10 Fingers for God* [a book about Dr. Paul Brand, who made monumental breakthrough in understanding leprosy. He grew up a missionary kid in India, suffering a range of local illnesses in his childhood.] I readily identified the Brands' child raising style as being very similar to my parents. 'I would rather a few of them died than any of them grow up to be wimps.' To their credit, our parents allowed us to grow up wild or free, depending on which way you look at it. The only two safety rules I can recall were 'Don't share spoons with any friend who is a TB patient.' 'No swimming after the generator comes on,' i.e., after dark."

Despite the lack of rules and the many NDE's—near death experiences—one thing was clear; the Calverts were loved and inherited an incredible foundation of faith from their parents. Their moral record, however, is not completely clear.

As children, their wildness did lead to petty crime. Hours of patience paid off as they fished pieces of copra—smoked coconut—through the floor slats to the store house. Later, they used these skills to get peacock feathers off the poor birds at aviaries in New Zealand. They also picked up on the "hunter-gatherer" skills of the area. Days were spent searching for mushrooms as well as raiding public hedges and road verges in search of edible fruit. If they weren't eating wild fruit and vegetables, they were hunting local animals. Bandicoots and sago grubs ranked at the top for most palatable choices. They did eat grasshoppers and beetles as well, but noted those were not nearly as tasty.

Ted said, "Kapuna is seasonal, wet or dry with a lot of rain falling in the dry season. Summer was for swimming, going on patrol, and playing games in the late afternoon and evenings. Winter was for roasting pumpkin seeds, manioc, and stale bread on the top of the wood stove. It was a Mecca for small boys towing any kind of boat in the flooded drains. It was also a Mecca for fungi. I had sleepless nights as the tine between my toes itched and drove me mad. Hallelujah for concrete paths that banished perpetual wet feet!"

Coastal PNG life is marked by life on the meandering rivers. It is no wonder that many of the childhood memories and near death experiences revolve around swimming and boating.

When Valerie was just three years old, the canoe that she and Dr. Peter were in broke down. Another boat came along to tow them. As soon as the rescue boat took off, the canoe immediately capsized. Valerie was grabbed out of the river by her father as she floated past. They made it safely to shore. Then, as a toddler, Ted wandered off and ended up in the water. Thankfully, a nurse was walking past and saw his blond head bobbing in the water. She fished him out just in time. From time to time, Dr. Lin would also peer out from their house and count the blond heads in the water, making sure all four were still afloat.

Youth in New Zealand were learning to drive their cars when the Calvert kids were becoming versed in navigating water crafts of many shapes, sizes, and speeds. While most of the travel in the area was done via canoe, a New Zealand acquaintance decided to donate a jet boat to the Calvert family. It was a lot of fun, but the jet boat was the source of many mishaps, several close calls for its passengers, and eventually its own demise. The main issue was that it was so fast its wake would capsize passing canoes if the driver was not attentive. One day, a visiting pastor had joined them for a boat ride to the villages. Alan was driving while the pastor and Ted, immersed in a book, were sitting on the boat. Logs and debris floating in the rivers were a constant hazard, especially for a speed boat. Too late, Alan noticed a large log blocking his path. In a panic, he accidentally accelerated rather than slowed. Hitting the log at a top speed, the boat went airborne and so did its passengers. Both Ted and the pastor were thrown into the water.

Logs, debris, and sandbars hidden in the water can wreak havoc on boats and outboard motors, if run over. In a similar jet boat incident, Ted was driving. Colin and Alan were enjoying the ride on the front of the boat when Ted took a corner too sharply. He overcorrected, landing directly on top of a sandbar, stopping the momentum of the boat. Both Colin and Alan were launched into the jungle landing not-so-gently in the foliage.

One of Ted's favorite jet boat memories was of it breaking down hours away from home on the river. He was on patrol with his father. His favorite radio show, to which he claimed he was addicted, was *The Muddled Headed Wombat and Captain Scarlet*. Taking the radio with him on patrol, Ted was unfazed when the jet boat broke down. The breakdown was just in time for him to tune into the program.

Needless to say, the adventures in the jet boat as well as the jet boat itself were short lived; it was not a very practical tool for PNG. It used too much fuel and caused too many close calls for its passengers and passing vessels.

Dr. Lin also shared memories of her life on the water. She and Peter were traveling back from New Zealand, visiting friends in the Solomon Islands on their way. This tropical paradise was enticing, so they borrowed a small boat on which to stay. Sleeping side by side in the open waters, she recalled the boat was not wide enough for them both to sleep on their backs. They had to rotate onto their sides for the other person to move. While it was a fond and memorable moment with her husband, they did not get much rest that way.

Water is an interwoven theme of coastal PNG as are the crocodiles and snakes that inhabit the rivers and swampy regions. My first trip to Papua New Guinea, on board the M/V Pacific Link, I remember sitting on the bow with a number of local guys scanning the water in search of the elusive crocodiles. We even jokingly threatened to use our friend Felix as bait.

PNG's animistic roots hold these creatures in high regard with godlike powers. It is no surprise then, that almost every person living in PNG has a number of memories associated with snakes and crocodiles.

"Challenges with snakes provided numerous memories throughout my years. Big long snakes with an enormous bulge revealed an elongated chicken or short ones dangling from a hen trying to swallow it. The only snakes we really feared were death adders as they didn't get out of the way. Proof of this was on a guava hunt to the old sawmill where five of us in single file stepped over an adder and it was only seen by the sixth child. We routinely killed snakes as we came across them," Ted said.

He described the moment his relationship with snakes officially changed. He and his friends noticed a snake sunning itself on the rooftop. Throwing sticks to dislodge it, they were successful. The snake dropped. Unfortunately, it dropped directly onto Ted's shoulders. I can only imagine the yells and appendage flailing that followed. After being flung off of Ted and slithering away into the tall grasses, I assume the snake developed the same dislike of teenage boys, as Ted now did of snakes.

The Calverts conveyed how Kapuna Hospital has seen a lot of victims of both snake and croc incidents. The mighty predator, the crocodile, is both hunter and hunted in the region. Many imprudent fortune hunters have traveled through seeking the beast for its skin, hoping to cash in on the bounty of these creatures in the area. One such victim had shot one. Rather than let the crocodile slip away, he jumped in the water after his presumed dead trophy. The crocodile was wounded but definitely not dead. The predictable ending landed the hunter in Kapuna hospital with bite wounds. Another fortune hunter never even made it to the crocodile. He smoked his cigarette while refueling his outboard motor. Needless to say, Kapuna has record of an explosion victim after that incident.

Like the other locals, the Calverts also grew up wielding machetes and hunting with bows and arrows.

"Wildness meant early use of axe and machete. We never got to the skill levels of our local friends but we were not too bad. My first machete was a Christmas present."

Machetes and axes were another product of colonization. These tools were traded or used as payment for services. Until the late 1700s, gardeners and hunters utilized stone axes and tools. I even purchased a stone ax from the markets in Port Moresby as a gift . . . More of a novelty now that metal is significantly easier to use.

In Kapuna one can see children as young as a few years old, wandering around with machetes. A trait not learned in school but in the daily life of the jungle, Papua New Guineans can cut, build, and prepare food with a few swings of a machete or axe. The incredible accuracy and strength in their skill is truly admirable.

There were a lot of priorities fostered while setting up a functioning hospital, as well as developing the area. A school would not emerge in Kapuna to meet the needs of the staff families until much later. It fell on Peter and Lin to home-school their four children in the midst of running a hospital. Dr. Lin held the honor of primary teacher and, of course, mother. School normally took place in the mornings since patrols and hospital rounds took up the afternoons. Many learning supplies were in short demand, so they improvised. They grew beans in jars and got creative for science experiments.

"Chemicals were hard to come by for experiments so I remember burning and crushing shells to get calcium. We also tried to 'explode' flour to show fine particles are more reactive than solid matter," Ted shared.

Their education was far from conventional. The greatest education, for all of them, was living life alongside their parents.

"We were forced into or given opportunities for leadership (depending on which way you look at it) from when we could walk and talk. This varied from acting in plays, helping dress sores on patrol, taking responsibility for equipment, or driving. My personal biggest tests were breaking up fights between adults when I was a pre-teen and I also was the driver when my passenger drowned after an accident." Ted did not expand much on the drowning story. Death is much more public and part of life in remote Papua New Guinea. Being a child of doctors, the Calvert children grew up with a more intimate understanding of this reality of life, than their New Zealand counterparts.

Knowing the homeschooling was only sufficient for so long, each kid left for high school in New Zealand when they hit about thirteen years old. Through it all, the Calvert family thrived. Valerie went on to become a doctor, both Ted and Alan pursued engineering, and Colin is now the hospital administrator and a huge advocate for development, leadership training, and Biblical training in the Purari Delta Region. They all highly value education. Throughout my time in Kapuna, Colin, Valerie, and Dr. Lin were all reading a variety of books, sharing with groups, running devotionals and teachings in the mornings. Many an evening around the dinner table they shared insight and wisdom.

Not only do they value education, the children have carried on their parent's faith. Through their incredible sacrifice, Peter and Lin laid a foundation of love and faith in their children.

This did not keep the children from testing the sanctity of visiting ministers. Since the local church, at the time, had a rotation of traveling missionary pastors, the Calvert kids favored some and were not very fond of others.

"Circuit ministers came in various shapes and sizes. We 'tormented' them or avoided them depending on their disposition. John Crib was the most famous and our favorite. While single, he was fair game for jokes and adventures, but after marriage, he mellowed a bit. He didn't completely calm down as he put baby crocodiles in his toddler's swimming pool and kept a python in his roof to deal with rats."

TRIALS OF BUILDING A HOSPITAL

While the Calvert children grew up with fond memories of life in PNG, it was not always an easy path, especially for Drs. Peter and Lin. Not every religious leader was in favor of the hospital; some even worked hard to have its progress stopped. Whether it was because of personal agendas, a tenacious clinging to tradition or resulting from negative experiences with previous ministries, there were many instances when Kapuna Hospital had opposition from religious groups and leaders.

New things, whether good or bad, tend to be met with opposition.

We heard one such tale around a bonfire one night.

Bec, Valerie's daughter-in-law, shouted from the ground that she was coming up. Our door was unlocked, so she pushed her way in and headed up the stairs to the main level of the little jungle house.

"Well, are you coming?" she asked.

"Where are we supposed to be going?" my roommate, Annaleigh, and I responded a little bit confused. Our usual quiet evening at home was being interrupted.

"Oh, I guess no one told you. We are having a fire and will be cooking damper behind Colin and Barb's house. You should come."

With not much else to fill our time after sunset, Annaleigh and I both jumped at the chance to socialize in a new setting. After all, evening chats with friends are a huge part of what made Papua New Guinea amazing!

We coated ourselves in another layer of mosquito spray, grabbed our house keys, and set off into the night.

The generators for Kapuna were still running. The dim lights from the houses melted through the vegetation, guiding our path on the narrow walkway. We followed that light over the slick bridges and around the hospital grounds. A few patients and caretakers still mingled on the porches; men clustered throughout the lawn, talking about the events of the day. A couple of local children, still out, greeted us and then giggled at each other for having the nerve to address a white-skin.

After we passed the church building, man-made lights gave way to the star-scattered indigo sky. We set out on a trampled path in the ankle deep grass expanding toward the pineapple patch. Just before the patch there stood a wide circle of palms. In the midst of them, we saw the blaze of a small campfire kept alive by burning coconut husks and shells. Dried palm leaves had been used as kindling.

It was serene as we settled on a fallen log; those joining us brought out chairs and a woven mat. Fresh into our conversation, my German friend and Kapuna volunteer, Gerald, jumped off of his seat, swatting at his midsection. My roommate and I soon followed.

Ants! These invasive, microscopic creatures were making their way into our clothing, biting quickly before our swats terminated their short lives. It is not unusual in the jungle to break into a flailing frenzy after large and small insects encroach on one's personal space. I had never better understood the term "ants in the pants" than after coming to PNG.

The others offered chairs or the woven mat as an alternative to our log. I settle on the woven mat with Bec and Barb.

Caleb, Valerie's son (Bec's husband), and Ted were preparing branches to put the damper on as we passed around bowls of fresh pineapple and papaya. I had grown up with marshmallows around campfires but had never experienced the doughy substance called damper until moving to Australia three years prior. It is a very basic mix of flour, water, and salt that is wrapped around sticks and cooked over an open fire. Once it is cooked and no longer pasty, one would pull it off the stick and smother it in butter, jam, honey, or other toppings.

That particular evening, some slapped the dough around the sticks hoping for best cooking techniques; others attempted more visual aesthetics by braiding and winding the damper into a work of art. Then, the branches were hovered over the embers and rotated from time to time.

I sat watching Gerald spend a frustrating amount of time trying to turn his damper into a pretzel with discouraging results. I motioned to him to pass his dough and stick to me. Skillfully, I reworked the dough. After wrapping it around the stick, he eyed it critically, "That looks exactly like what I just did."

I laughed. It really wasn't much better. I never was good with sculpture.

Laughter, good natured teasing, and conversation flowed.

Ted finished his damper first. Quickly removing the piping hot dough from the stick, he bragged about its perfection as he spread jam across it.

Bec chimed in, "Uncle Colin, tell us a miraculous story from Kapuna."

Colin leaned in, placing his elbows on his knees. He was pensive for a few moments. What incredible story could he tell? There were so many that took place here.

A slow smile spread across his face as he remembered. So began his tale of the bishop who tried to shut down the hospital.

In the 1970s, Christian revival, defined as a time of reawakened religious activity, had been spreading around the region, bringing with it unconventional ideas and practices for the time. The traditional church felt it was being challenged.

Because the revival had sprung out of Kapuna, the long standing religious leaders in the area were growing concerned. Some had received inaccurate reports of what was going on, so the church sent a bishop to check it out and put a stop to the hospital and work being done.

The bishop, a heavy smoker, had a long journey ahead of him as he traveled through the coastal terrain. While he made his way to Kapuna, the locals had received word he was coming and began to earnestly pray for God to intervene.

Traversing the swamp, the unlucky bishop was soon impeded by a large thorn in his foot. The tropical climate is rarely kind to injuries. Infection and swelling were imminent. The poor bishop! By the time his canoe arrived at the jetty in Kapuna he was on a stretcher, in extreme pain, and struggling to catch his breath.

Rather than shut down the hospital, he was carried in and admitted.

After days of receiving incredible care, he decided the hospital was necessary to the area. Taking his leave, he thanked the staff. Years later, he returned, bringing gifts and kind words with him.

As Uncle Colin wrapped up the story, we all smiled. Over thirty years later, we see more clearly just how miraculous the impact of Kapuna is. Imagining this patch of jungle without Kapuna seems daunting. After all what would so many people do without this hospital?

We could not help having a bit of sympathy for the the bishop, all knowing full well the harshness of the bush, yet we are grateful to see the results of the hospital in our current day having long since expanded into the lifeblood of this community. Of course, the church in mention now has an excellent relationship with Kapuna.

THE CHURCH

Peter and Lin were not just doctors. They were very much involved in the local church and community. Eventually, they felt led away from the traditional Western Church ways that the missionaries kept bringing. They realized a lot of the practices were merely traditions built around a different culture and wanted to see a church sprout up with local authenticity, training leaders and allowing people to participate rather than spectate. The Calverts desired all willing members to preach, teach, or help with music. To this day, there is no official pastor. Each Sunday, someone different in the community or a visitor shared from Scripture.

Dr. Lin wrote about this aspect of their lives in her book, *Let the Fire Burn*.

Many years ago, as Peter and I well-remembered, several churches in PNG, including our own, were planning to unite. One senior missionary suggested that instead of having a statement of doctrine and a constitution, we simply agree: "Jesus is Lord of this church." His wise advice, if followed, would have saved years and years of arguments! This simple confession of faith has proved completely adequate, not only for the Kapuna Fellowship, but also for all the other fellowships that have arisen in villages touched by the revival. Up until today they have continued without any divisions or arguments whatsoever over points of doctrine.

We have often had to list the important differences between these fellowships and a typical church congregation, and I feel this list may be helpful to others. Each difference is, we believe, a move nearer to the type of group Jesus planned to be His Body on earth.

1. There is no permanent leadership. Leaders arise as the need arises. If a leader falls away or moves away, another unobtrusively takes over the leadership. As a rule, decisions are made by the whole group, they are made by discussion and prayer rather than by voting. This fits PNG traditional thinking very well.

2. Funds are raised and spent on the initiative of the group. Most of their money is used to buy petrol to visit other fellowships. Leaders are not paid. They all belong to the villages where they are acting as leaders.

3. Believer's baptism, Spirit baptism, deliverance, laying hands on the sick, and anointing with oil are all an essential part of every group's ministry.

4. No titles are used; everyone is addressed as "brother" or "sister."

5. At worship services, all are encouraged to share, join in the group prayers, bring a teaching, a song, a dream or vision, an experience or a testimony. There is much emphasis on the importance of sharing, because only in this way is every Christian encouraged. It is sad that in a traditional

service the leader in particular often feels no one prayed for his special needs.

6. There is much emphasis on the importance of forgiveness. All are encouraged to solve their problems before coming to the fellowship meeting. Frequently, we have someone waiting at the entrance who will question believers about this. The discipline of the fellowship members is in the hands of the whole Christian group, not of the leaders. If a group let their fellowship die through undealt-with sins, we do give advice if asked, but we do not insist on any particular course of action being followed. It is God's family, not ours.

7. Some fellowships have agreed to keep certain rules they have decided on for themselves, e.g., no pagan funeral customs, no lucky charms, no betel nut chewing, no smoking, and so on.

PETER'S DEATH

In the early 1980s, Peter discovered that he had an enlarged liver. The bowel cancer which was removed earlier had returned. He fought a brave battle against the disease, holding out as long as he could against each stage of it. Always he encouraged the rest of Kapuna in every aspect of the work, both Christian and medical.

Dr. Lin shared how he tenaciously clung to his faith, "Two church leaders came to visit him about a month before he died. They invited him to apologize for his part in the revival but he refused to take the opportunity. He told them, 'All my life I have been happy but these last few years have been the happiest of all. It is the Holy Spirit who brought revival here. How can I apologize for His work or for letting me be part of it?'"

Peter was confident into his death. When sad orderlies came to see him, he encouraged them, telling them to smile because he knew he was destined for Heaven.

Dr. Lin said, "We called Valerie and her husband, Bryan, on the radio. A Mission Aviation Fellowship pilot, in a wonderful gesture of kindness, brought the whole family straight down from Mt. Hagen where they had gone for a brief trip. The weather was wet and the air strip was closed but the chief pilot came down himself and the strip was opened for an emergency landing. They reached home while Peter was still strong enough to pray with the seven of us, one by one. We watched beside him all night but he did not leave us then. In the morning he was still conscious but his voice had faded to a faint whisper as he said 'I'm so thankful they came last night. I couldn't have said goodbye to them today.'"

Dr. Peter died at Kapuna, July 23, 1982. In her book, Dr. Lin wrote of his death and funeral. Peter was PNG at heart, and in PNG his body would stay.

> We buried him near the baptism creek, a place he dearly loved to go. He never missed a baptism if he could help it. Hundreds came from the two nearby villages. Some even chartered a plane from Kerema and arrived in time for the funeral, though this was held the same day that he died. All of us praised his life and prayed that our lives might be as fruitful and effective as his had been. Village leaders and many others took the chance to say thank you to the Lord for his life of service. Nobody wailed, nobody cried. How could we cry on the day that the one we all loved had received his victory crown? Valerie, in a vision, actually saw him having it placed on his head!

> Peter had told me more than once, 'If I should die at Kapuna, I want the bush to grow over my grave.' So we would allow no cement or headstone, just frangipani and hibiscus, crotons and the red leaves used for dressing up at celebrations. A nearby fellowship asked permission to put a wooden railing all around it and we agreed to this. We ourselves held a picnic close by soon after he died, and later the nurses decided to make their gardens there. Locally all

the traditional thoughts and teachings on death seemed to have been turned upside down just because Peter chose to die among the people he served. As far as I know he is one of the very few modern missionaries in PNG to die and be buried at his place of work. How natural and peaceful and right it all seemed.

There were times I wished I could have met Dr. Peter and heard of his life first hand. But, after seeing where Kapuna Hospital is thirty years after his death and meeting his devoted children and grandchildren, I realize, I have seen his legacy, the fruit of this man's work.

THE CALVERTS TODAY

Each Calvert child returned to New Zealand, one at a time to finish school. Valerie was the first to go. Physically, the petite blond mirrors her mother in looks and very much in personality. She followed her parents on the path to medicine. In fact, in the 1970s, Valerie studied medicine in Port Moresby where she met Bryan Archer, a New Zealand builder, who was working on various projects throughout the city.

They were married and had four children, two daughters and two sons. She spent most of her time in New Zealand raising their family and working. Of course, Kapuna was a part of their history and their kids built many memories around the bush hospital. Valerie returned to work at the hospital after her marriage ended. She recognized Kapuna was ingrained in her DNA and her mother needed another hand at the hospital.

Both Ted and Alan married and settled into work as engineers. True to their upbringing, however, their families also spent a good portion of their lives in PNG. Both brothers used their skill to do development work for Kapuna. Ted returns annually for at least a month to help with logistics and important paperwork. Although he claims retirement, like his mother and sister, that means very little as he continues to work all over the world, lending his engineering skills to many international humanitarian projects.

Colin had stuck by his mother's side while his father battled cancer. In his father's absence, he helped to oversee and run the hospital. He eventually returned to New Zealand to attend Faith Bible College, where he met a stunning, dark haired, green eyed Kiwi girl, Barbara. She shared his faith, adventurous nature, and willingly followed him back to Kapuna after they were married. Together they built a life much like his parents in Kapuna. Colin and Barb run the hospital administration, along with discipleship training, many local church functions, and now the local school.

In Kapuna, they had five bright and creative children, tragically losing one as an infant. After the death of a good friend and fellow staff member, Colin and Barb adopted her daughter, Stephanie. Stephanie was a natural fit as a close friend to their daughters.

A TALE OF TWO GRANDMOTHERS

The machete and long, hooked knife lean up against the wall in the bathroom (the same bathroom I found a live rat in the previous week). The initials "DR" for doctor scratched into the handle were almost worn away with time. If anyone could guess the owner, they would probably not associate them with a tiny 89-year-old New Zealand woman.

"Grandma," as everyone lovingly calls Dr. Lin Calvert, is absolutely nothing like the grandma I grew up with. The contrasts are almost astounding. While both Dr. Lin and my grandma were petite, striking women with white hair and sun-kissed skin, the similarities end there.

I had the joy of living with my 89-year-old grandmother when I was in my early twenties. Her spotless home still had its original 1970s brown or olive green flowered wallpaper. Her decorations were collected from all over the world; she and my grandfather had taken exotic trips to places like Fiji and Panama. They had always stayed in comfortable cruise-liner cabins, mingling only in specific local markets, taking in the touristy sights.

I loved that house full of good-cooking smells. Even though a bit outdated, it was a super stylish and immaculately clean home, much like my grandmother.

After two hip surgeries, she still insisted on wearing high heels everywhere. Since early childhood, I remember her constantly painted red toenails and her standing hair appointment every Friday. Her white/blonde hair went well with her blue eyes and red lipstick. My grandmother was beautiful and loved beautiful things.

While I look nothing like her, I did inherit a love of beauty and making things around me beautiful and homey—no matter where I am in the world.

The other thing I inherited from my grandmother is her love of reading. I cannot count the amount of nights I found her sound asleep in her chair, a book open across her chest, and the reading light still on. My mom does the exact same thing. I do the exact same thing. So many times I've awoken in the middle of the night, picked myself up off the couch, removed the open book from my chest, and gone to bed. We get into books and cannot put them down.

In stark contrast, I walked past the markets in Kapuna, Papua New Guinea the other day and had to do a double take. There was Grandma Lin in gumboots, standing in a drainage ditch with her thin arms, swinging a machete. Her wheelbarrow was piled high with weeds as she cleared the ditch on a hot, sunny afternoon. She was still very much the New Zealand farm girl.

Her minimalistic clapboard home serves as the main office building, as well as a gathering place in the mornings for devotionals and hymn singing. Sitting on a creaky metal bed-frame covered in faded quilts or with folded legs on the grey-ing wood floor, Kapuna students and staff raise their voices in ancient hymns or local songs with Grandma Lin knowing every word by heart. A few feet away in her open doorway, a large dented aluminum bowl holds crumbled sago drying in the harsh tropical sun.

Pinned on the faded walls are photos of family, a black-and-white portrait of a young, smiling Dr. Peter and Dr. Lin, and a few staff weddings.

Once songs end, I can hear Grandma Lin's raspy Kiwi accent reading from a missionary's history or the Bible.

This little old doctor is strong and resilient. With her husband buried in the area, she continues to work amongst the people she loves.

But, more than anything, she is a woman of deep faith. Sometimes, as I walk past her office, I stand still for a while, gazing at her diminutive frame bent over her Bible. Her thick white hair is clipped back the way she wore it in the 60s. With a sweater over her thin shoulders and thick warm wool socks on her feet, she finds the tropics chilly. Grandma Lin is stunning. To the right of her Bible is a notepad scribbled full of notes and memories of things God has taught her throughout her life.

She is a woman so deeply in love with God, she not only endured life in the harsh jungle, but thrived in it, carving out a place of beauty and healing. Like my grandma, she loves beautiful things. Unlike my grandma, Dr. Lin finds it in her tropical garden and in her love of her patients in the weather worn bush hospital.

It makes me think deeply about the legacy I will one day leave. I pray my grandchildren (and anyone willing to call me Grandma) can look in admiration and say, "Now there is a woman who loves God."

Thanks for the life lessons, Grandma and Grandma!

COMMUNITY HEALTHCARE WORKER SCHOOL

Another feature of Kapuna is their training facility. For over fifty years, Kapuna has had a two-year Community Healthcare Worker (CHW) training course, followed by a six month internship.

Both male and female students from all over Papua New Guinea receive classroom and hands-on training at Kapuna Hospital. Throughout the semester, they are sent for practicals in surrounding villages. At their village placements, the students put into practice their recent education which entails community assessment projects, hygiene, health education, and clinics.

Due to so many remote, hard-to-reach places in PNG, CHWs are vital to the health and well-being of much of PNG's population. The trained healthcare workers are placed throughout villages and in hard to reach places. This system has been around since World War II. In essence, the CHW provides Primary Health Care in areas with limited to no access to hospitals or doctor's offices. Their training covers a wide range of medical issues. Despite it only being a two year school, many CHWs are faced with monumental challenges in the field. Many times they refer severe cases to the hospitals, but since they can be hours or days away, they may be required to do their best to stabilize patients and make immediate decisions for care.

The school takes on about twenty new students each year. They arrive from all over the nation after testing and selection to attend. Classes are rigorous, tackling a vast range of topics.

Shy Lucy and her husband, Bob, both PNG nationals, head the school. Just a few weeks prior to my arrival, Lucy had been stricken by a mysterious illness and almost died. She told of her miraculous recovery the day I met her, my first Sunday in church.

In her resilience, she improved quickly. As her closest neighbor, daily I saw her working in her garden, swinging a machete to rid weeds and unwanted growth and yet delicately handling the beautiful flower buds. Lucy has a gift for nurturing life. She hardly says a word and smiles at her feet, yet her love is palpable.

Bob is less shy. He has a full beard and an even fuller good nature with a big smile shining through.

Through Bob and Lucy's guidance, along with the teaching of the doctors, the students acquire a lot of knowledge in two short years. They also join Grandma Lin for story time and Bible studies, attend classes, and then meet with the staff on ward rounds to get hands-on experience.

Kapuna would not be the same without the students. Not only do they help in several ways at the hospital, they always seem to find time for a good laugh or guitar music. Several nights I drifted to sleep as clear voices harmonized to a guitar, drifting from the guys' dorm. They also found time for sports. A field on the outskirts of Kapuna houses countless past and present rugby matches. The blood and sweat of many CHW student has been spilt on that field in good-natured competition. Rugby, the fantastically fast-paced and brutal game, is a favorite amongst British Commonwealth and Pacific Islands. I would watch from a distance, envious that it was only culturally appropriate in Kapuna for men to play. After all my years in Australia I was drawn into learning and loving the sport.

The school is such a natural fit for a hospital whose desire is multiplication. Sustainability is a key factor in developing the Baimuru region and the Gulf Province. The best results for a lasting, positive impact is through community.

Kapuna has strong ties to the local community. The Calverts know that you cannot merely treat physical symptoms of people and a region, so Kapuna strives to educate and lead by example.

Throughout the year, the staff and students go to neighboring villages for outreaches. These involve hands-on learning, clinics, teaching, as well as getting to know the locals.

They also run a number of programs from Kapuna, including: field days for the kids, World AIDS Day awareness teaching, parenting classes, and healthy village "ene vapara."

"Ene vapara" or healthy village is run throughout the area for week long teachings. It helps the locals better understand illnesses and how to recognize what should be done in each situation; breaking down long-held cultural beliefs about sickness and its causes; educating locals on preventative measures is fundamental to healthy villages.

The long-term goal of "Ene vapara" is to see a first-aid kit and thermometer in the hands of each mother, as well as the skill to best utilize the tools.

SURVIVING THE JUNGLE: VARAE AND THE SAGO SWAMP

My first night in Kapuna was rough. Enclosed in my mozzie net, the warm air was stifling. I had finally drifted off only to be awoken by the chickens laying eggs or the bats getting into the nearby fruit trees. The frogs in the nearby swamp were the worst. I would eventually grow accustomed to the sounds of the jungle, but not that night. Rising with the sun, my body was damp from sweating in the foam mattress.

Annaleigh and I enjoyed a quick breakfast and coffee on our deck before church. She was great company. We had known each other less than a day and we were fast friends, laughing together.

Two tall, lean men with curly mops of hair and full beards passed. They must be the New Zealand school builders, I thought. We called down to them. They paused and smiled up at us. I thought they must be brothers at first. Introducing themselves as Brooke and Simon, I found out they were just best friends. They excused themselves as they headed to the Treehouse where Caleb and Bec, Dr. Valerie's family, were staying. Visitors are only common in this area if they serve a purpose and come for at least a few months. Kapuna's remoteness and the inconsistency of transportation make it pointless otherwise. Simon, an old friend of Bec's, and Brooke agreed to join her and Caleb last minute. The original builders arranged to help the locals build a new school cancelled their trip without much notice.

We then joined Gerald on his way to church. The bell had rung about thirty minutes earlier, but since this was Papua New Guinea, we knew most people would not show up for at least an hour. They filtered slowly in.

It did not take long to learn a church service in Papua New Guinea had no set time limit. The gathering was also a way to catch up with events and people. So much of it involved announcements and people sharing tales of recent travels or things going on in their lives. My rear tingled with numbness from sitting for hours on the wood floor with the locals. I had not thought to bring a fan that first day, so I wiped my damp forehead with my sleeve throughout the service.

After a quick lunch with the guys and Annaleigh at the Treehouse, Caleb announced we were going on a varae hunt! It was a rare, flowering fruit found at the base of trees in the swamp. Prior to lunch, Caleb taught Brooke, Simon, and I how to husk a coconut on the sharp stick, crack it open, and scrape it out. The guys became concerned I may impale myself as I threw down all of my body weight in an effort to get the husk off the coconut. It was a full-body effort. I never did master it, relying on locals or Annaleigh to handle my coconut prep.

Simon, Brooke, Caleb, Isaka, and a few of the students joined me on the hunt. Donning red floral gumboots, baggy cotton pants, and a sweat stained shirt, I was a fashionable sight to see. Wielding machetes, we followed single file into the swamp behind our garden. Pausing to check a bandicoot trap, we were stunned by electrifying pain all over our bodies. Huge red ants invaded our clothing. We had to keep moving.

As we trudged in further, the mud became deeper and more intense. I started to sink. The next step took me down further and my gumboots were completely stuck. Caleb pulled me out. A few steps later, I was stuck again. I started to learn to step from tree debris to tree debris rather than just anywhere. Each time I sank, ants swarmed up my legs, biting relentlessly. Sweat poured down my back.

The vegetation cleared for us to see a massive sago swamp. These special palms had long, dangerous thorns. Legend goes that the natives found sago was good for eating when they watched wild pigs dig into the palms with their tusks, eating the interior. Once felled, sago is hollowed out with axes and hoes. The insides are then turned into pulp, beaten with sticks at a sago stand, sifted, and then water is run through it. The drain-off from the water and fine pulp is collected. It congeals and hardens into blocks. A person takes chunks of it off the block as needed. The block crumbles easily and is then cooked in several different ways. This starchy, bland diet is the main food staple for coastal Papua New Guineans.

It is grueling work, made dangerous by the swamp and long spikes.

Varae is also found in this swamp. Caleb plucked up a few. A white, layered flower with red highlights peeled open to reveal dark seeds. If the seeds are still white, they are not ready to eat and very tart. Popping a bunch of the tiny, crunchy seeds into my mouth, I was pleasantly surprised. It was one of the sweetest fruits I had tasted, reminding me of a slightly sour berry. They warned us not to enjoy too many since they constipate.

After gathering several varae, we made our way out of the swamp. I felt a little better about myself after I watched one of the CHW students tumble out of his yellow gumboots and fall face first into the mud. At least I was not the only clumsy one.

We navigated our way back through a garden where the guys stopped to machete a few sugar canes. Chewing on stalks, we emerged sweaty, dirty, and bitten, but happy. If I were keeping score it would be: Jungle 1, White-skin female 0.

Thankfully, a cold, rainwater shower awaited my return and soothed my bitten skin.

GOOD MORNING, PNG

The rooster crowed again. One further away answered back. Then in unison, rooster sounds rose, filling the air. It was like they were in competition with each other, each wanting to be just a bit more obnoxious than the last.

I flung my bed sheet aside, unclipped the clothes pegs holding my mosquito net shut, and pitched myself out of bed. My patience had expired. I rubbed my bleary eyes and looked out the window. The sun was barely up, signifying it was still very early morning in the tropics.

Stupid *grumble* roosters!

I had never purposely killed an animal in my life, but I was on the verge of homicidal thoughts towards those feathered creatures. My bush diet severely lacked protein; the roosters would be wise not to tempt me.

I considered going back to bed and putting in my headphones, but I was already sweating from the heat and humidity. My mattress just seemed to envelope my damp skin, heating it up more.

No. A cold shower and coffee were what I needed. I shuffled into the kitchen, grabbed the kettle, and stood with it in my hands for a while. My dim mental faculties were not capable of deciding whether to start with the coffee or the shower. I eventually set the empty kettle back down and turned toward the stairs.

Shower it is.

Halfway down the stairs I brushed the sticky spider web out of my face before continuing.

Squeeeeeee

I pushed the bathroom door open and as always it made a horrific creaking noise. I made a quickly forgotten mental vow that I would find a way to oil that door.

Squeeeeeee

It swung shut behind me.

Shower time. I took off my sweaty pajamas and stepped into the shower. The wisdom in a tropical shower is to check your surroundings before stepping in. Almost every form of jungle insect had managed to die during the night in the small pool of water at the bottom of the shower or was alternatively stuck to the wall, maimed, fighting for its last hold on life. Why they all came to our bathroom for the end of their lives, I will never know.

Due to my semiconscious state, I cared less than normal about all of the insect life (or lack thereof) and stepped into the shower.

Dammit!

Half dead cricket got stuck to the bottom of my foot. It was definitely dead now. I tried scraping it off to no avail, so I turned on the shower.

Ahhhhhh!

The cold water cascaded down my chest. I grabbed my washcloth and proceeded to do the cold water hokey-pokey. Just like it sounds, one bit of my body at a time went under the icy deluge until all of me was rinsed and clean. At this point of the shower, my body temperature adjusted and I put my head under.

Propping my forehead against the wall, I let it run down my back for a while. Go figure the only thing cold in coastal Papua New Guinea is the shower.

SMACK!

I smashed a mosquito against the wall, but not before it proceeded to add a few more itchy bumps to my body. I turned off the water after rinsing a few more dead bugs down the drain.

By the time I had finished toweling off, sweat was beading on my skin again. *Sigh* So much for no stains on the clean shirt today. I stepped out of the bathroom to head back upstairs for my coffee, but not before stepping on a few more dead insects and walking through a fresh spider's web.

I started the kettle on our gas burner and grabbed my blue bag of Goroka coffee—only this coffee snob's favorite coffee on the planet.

"Thank you, Jesus, for creating coffee," I prayed out of gratitude as I inhaled deeply from the package before dumping the contents into my press. While waiting for the water to boil, I checked for bread. My options for breakfast were bread or bread but only if we make it the night before. Otherwise, digging for leftovers or making a bowl of two minute noodles are the options.

Bread it is! I opened the bread maker to see if our loaf had risen. Half the time, it is small and spongy. The reason for the random bread not rising is a mystery, yet we eat it because it's what we have.

Taking my piping hot cup of java and bread doused in the hot sauce I brought with me, I sat on my deck and looked out over the carpet of jungle vegetation. I sighed a content sigh. At that moment, I loved my life. I couldn't believe I got to wake up in PNG. I thought to myself, "Bring on the day!"

I scratched a few more mosquito bites, wiped my sweat moustache, and enjoyed my morning.

ANNALEIGH

For three weeks I shared the little bush house with Annaleigh, also known as AJ. She was a complete anomaly in this bush setting. New Zealand born and raised, she was close to her big family, an accomplished dancer with heaps of brains: a Business Degree in management, as well as a BA in Development Studies and International Relations. My favorite thing about AJ, however, was her contagious laugh. She could see the bright side of just about anything.

We howled hysterically as she told me how she ended up in Kapuna. Soon after finishing her long stint at University, she followed her friend Emma and her husband, out to Kapuna for a six week visit. Annaleigh had come to support her friends who were on the brink of moving to Kapuna as volunteers. Soon after returning to New Zealand from her visit, it was she, not her friends, who Kapuna Hospital pursued. They needed her business acumen in their office for paperwork, bookkeeping, and accounts.

Driving around Wellington with tears streaming down her face, she argued with God and even swore a little, knowing what her answer was going to be in the end.

The stylish, young Kiwi woman moved to the swamp and so began her two year journey. Battling loneliness, culture shock, as well as bugs and rodents, AJ carved out a place here, all the while seeing it through the bright eyes of her humorous disposition.

She immediately took me in, teaching me the ways of the jungle. She would husk coconuts for me; I would crack and scrape them in return. Since she returned to New Zealand frequently, she also had a stash of chocolate and cheese that she rationed out and shared with those of us who were less prepared.

Recently, AJ made the hard decision to return to New Zealand. Her two-year mark on Kapuna, however, would not be quickly forgotten. Forsaking just about everything she knew in her 20-something life, she had persevered in the bush. She also managed to turn the Kapuna elementary students into the best dancers the Gulf Province could ask for.

My favorite AJ moment was when she donned bright yellow gum boots, a long sleeved shirt, and a machete. Determined to tame the bush, I listened to her hacking away at the overgrowth in the garden out back. Shrieks soon followed. She came rushing into the house, a swarm of bees in hot pursuit. In her jungle clearing, she had disturbed a nest. I tried to sympathize but I was paralyzed with laughter. Poor, swollen, stung, unfortunate AJ. As usual, the PNG bush won.

NIGHT ON THE RIVER

The distant lightning split the night sky. Our surroundings lit up in a glow. We could make out the silhouette of the towering palms with the billowing storm clouds illuminated. It was so distant we could barely hear the roll of thunder. The stars scattered across the Southern Hemisphere's sky. We spotted Orion, hardly making out the constellations for the brilliancy of the night.

The Wame River lay completely still. Its broad banks were only disturbed by the ripples from our aluminum boat as we cut through the murky water. The river was an almost perfect mirror. A slightly hazy view turned upside down.

There was no electricity or unnatural light diminishing our surroundings. On a rare occasion, we would come across an ever increasing glow of a fire burning in a village along the shores, but it quickly melted into the trees as we passed.

The night air was tranquil. If we stopped the outboard motor, all was still, almost stifling.

The majority of the changes made in this area were carved out by the river's path. Otherwise, the landscape was a replica of what existed hundreds of years ago. It was one of the unchanged, expected things in this Land of the Unexpected.

It was awe inspiring.

We had started our journey not in search of beauty, but in pursuit of the mighty crocodile. As I climbed into the boat, I stepped over a harpoon with a rope attached to its end. Night time was the best for finding this scary creature whose strength and cunning had terrified the people of this region.

No greater predator was to be found. Many of the locals had stories of death resulting from this beast and his pursuit. We had probably passed many during our boat rides on the Wame but never saw them so skillfully disguised in their surroundings. The crocodiles came out at night, nesting in the muddy banks as the tide rolled in with the phases of the moon.

Not long after we had started our journey from Kapuna's banks, we spotted glowing specks that danced in the sky and skimmed the water's surface.

Fireflies!

They, too, were creatures of the night, only the contrast was extreme. They were delicate, traveled en mass, and bold, unlike the shy and powerful croc.

Our eyes followed the first few fireflies that showed themselves. As we traced their dancing pattern, they drew our gaze to the mangrove trees along the banks. The result took our breath away as millions of these glowing insects filled the mangroves, illuminating the entire tree. It was impossible to focus on a small cluster; we took in the full effect.

We killed the motor and drifted under the mangrove.

Due to the darkness of the night combined with the illumination of the tree, our world became surreal. The effect made us feel weightless; the tiny, elusive lights danced around us.

We shook a few branches and were showered in the fragile glow.

We continued our journey turning down smaller tributaries. Our spotlight resumed scanning the muddy banks for the crocodiles.

From time to time, we would pass another lit up mangrove. The spotlight would quickly scatter the bugs; the effect was a dispersing of light into the night sky.

In the silence of the night, tears began to fill my eyes. I marveled at the creation surrounding me. From the far-off flashes of lightening to the strength of the magnificent crocodile to the intricate glow of the firefly, I was sitting in indescribable splendor. The beauty was astounding.

Sometimes our greatest gifts are the unexpected. PNG was etched upon my heart in a new way. So often in my Western thinking, I understood the unexpected to be a negative trait. Here in this adventure, unexpected exceeded anything I could anticipate.

It reminded me in the midst of my ponderings on an unknown future, that I had a God who created all of this. He gave cunning and strength to the crocodile. He gave the firefly enchantment to dwell in the mangrove. He gave me beauty that night. Through the ripples in the water and reflection of the night sky, He reminded me that all of this creation, the very idea of beauty was created just for me to minister to my heart and remind me of His great love.

We never found any crocodiles, yet it was the most fruitful crocodile hunt one could be on.

I had no words, only tears. It was an overflow of a full heart, a grateful heart.

KIKIRAPU

"You have got to be kidding me! You want me to eat what?"

Kikirapu! The giant maggot looking creature sat in Caleb's hand only inches from my face. It is also known as a sago grub. *Kikirapu* makes its home in the sago trees which are a main part of the coastal Papua New Guinean diet, so naturally it, too, is a component of PNG nourishment.

I looked at the grub. Looked at Caleb. Looked back at Gerald, Simon, and Brooke sitting behind him. They all nodded with smiles. The four of them assured me they had just tried it. Caleb had grown up in PNG, of course he was okay with it.

"But, I did not get to watch you eat yours. I don't feel like this is completely fair."

No sympathy.

My protests fell on deaf ears.

Caleb handed me a small one. I stared at the cooked white maggot creature. I had eaten a tarantula when I was in Cambodia, surely I could put this in my mouth. Ugh! But, it was a giant maggot, essentially. My mind dissented, but I was never one to back down from a challenge.

I opened my mouth and dropped him in. A crunch followed by chewing. And more chewing. And more chewing!

This stupid grub would not break down in my mouth. The taste was like a terribly rancid nut.

I finally succeeded in swallowing it and pounding back a swig of coffee. Yuck!

The guys were laughing. I think my face said more than anything I could express.

Then, Caleb handed me a stick of sago with *kikirapu* packed into it.

"Have a bite. You need to experience it in the sago like the locals eat it."

The heavy aftertaste was still lingering in my mouth as I held this sago stick packed full of grubs. As quickly as I could, I bit off a section with two. The chewing again! It was so rubbery and so repulsive.

The more I thought about what I was eating, the more I could not swallow. Come on, little guys, you have got to go down.

I gagged.

I swallowed.

I clawed at the closest cup near me as I gasped for air. Dumping coffee down my throat again, I tried to rinse out the flavor. No words, just horror. My American palate was not ready for the rawness or the uniqueness of the jungle diet.

In typical American fashion, I handled it like any great exaggerated drama. My British friends would have kept a stiff-upper-lip and chalked it up to a new experience. For the rest of the day, I could taste this "delicacy" of the coastal lands.

A few days later when the guys brought me back some live ones from the bush, I resolutely declined. The grubs slimed their way across my plate. Once was enough.

I had felt a little bad about my response until I watched Annaleigh gag on one and spit it out.

No, I had made the right decision. Sorry, PNG, you can keep your *kikirapu*.

ISLAND TIME AND TERMITES

I had just turned on my computer and was waiting for programs to load. The office windows let in the warm breeze and roosters' noise. I was the first one in the office, having come in early, inspired to spend my uninterrupted morning writing. Planning in the Land of the Unexpected seemed futile, however. All illusions of productivity dissipated as Bec popped her head around the corner. A lovely smile lit up her face.

"Are you coming to Baimuru?" she asked.

"Baimuru? I had no idea anyone was going to Baimuru," I said a bit confused but not surprised. Communication was a seemingly lost art.

"This morning they decided they needed to take some lumber back for the school building. Apparently it was really bad wood, we need to get a replacement from the mill."

While I had a lot to do, I had been craving Coke and wanting to check the markets for garlic and onions, a rare but necessary cooking staple for the bland, starchy bush food. I also really admired Bec and wanted to spend more time chatting with her.

I grabbed my bag and money, following her to the large aluminum canoe. We had been informed the vessel was leaving immediately. In island time, that could mean any time in the next hour or so. Sunscreen applied, umbrella in hand, we sat on the floor of the boat and waited. Bec had not left Levi, her baby boy, for very long and was contemplating taking him. Torn, she wrestled with knowing we would likely be gone much longer than promised by the driver.

His round face and tuft of sweaty, orange hair sticking up in every direction appeared in the arms of Anna, one of the Kapuna staff. She was reveling in carrying the chubby, white skinned baby around. Bec leapt from her spot and ran after Anna. Taking Levi for just a few minutes while we waited for departure, she snuggled him and nursed.

A few patients climbed on board with their possessions in dilapidated plastic luggage. Toting her precious cargo, a new mum stepped onto the skive, intermittently, cautiously glancing with pride at the tiny person in her arms.

Eventually, everyone was settled onboard; sweat was beading as we sat in the stagnant jetty air waiting for the outboard to kick to life. The driver revved it a few times. Hesitantly, Bec handed Levi back to his caretaker and we made our way onto the Wame River. Rounding bend after bend of the river, we headed back the way I had arrived just weeks earlier. Every time I thought we were close or that I recognized the pervasive jungle vegetation, we took a different turn. My sense of direction was completely baffled throughout the trip.

With legs crossed, bags in hand, Bec and I sat that the bottom of the canoe, shifting from time to time to keep from losing circulation. I finally had my chance to learn a lot about her incredible life story. Just a few years my senior, she was one of those women who portrayed a natural and captivating beauty that ran much deeper than her exterior. I was riveted, listening to her account of meeting Caleb and their life around the world together. Tales of Nigeria and Indonesia filled our time.

I could see the teeming African city, spread out in my imagination, with its noisy traffic and tall apartments. Then, the motos and smells of street vendors filled my senses as she shared about raising two small children in Indonesia. I was encouraged that living internationally and having a family did not need to be mutually exclusive. Her innate sense of adventure was evident through her tales.

Our kindred spirits bonded.

Rather than head to Baimuru once we reached the river intersection, we turned left. Stopping off at random clearings with villages peeping through, one by one, patients were dropped off. The new mother, clutching her infant in one arm and bag of worldly possessions in the other, skillfully scaled a narrow log. Lithely, she made her way up a few more planks and onto the banks. An older woman briefly greeted her, holding out her arms for the baby. Once the baby was securely in her arms, the matron disappeared ahead of the new mother into the village.

Next, we arrived at a village where an elderly man with a harsh cough seated at the back of the canoe was greeted onshore by his family. They ran off, emerging ten minutes later with fresh fruit, a change of clothing, and some bedding for him. The children, in the meantime, showed off by jumping into the water, splashing each other and laughing.

A few more of these hospital drop-offs or pick-ups took place. The driver turned us back up river. Drifting past the first landing at the Chinese store, we landed next to the Baimuru station. Bec and I stepped off, walking across floating timber and finally stepping onto soggy saw dust and mud.

Joe, the station manager, greeted us with his wide grin showing gaps where many teeth were missing. Tribal tattoos covered his brown arms but his once imposingly large Maori stature was now a bit soft from years of office work. He was friendly and even more excited to find out Bec hailed from his native New Zealand. Justin, my inbound flight friend, joined us outside their office building to chat. Our driver went off to drop the bad timber and pick up the replacements.

Patience. A lesson I was bound to learn over and over again in PNG. Bec and I were offered a dinghy ride over to the tiny shop to get some cold, fizzy drinks. The sun was glaring overhead and hot now. We were both hungry, as well, but had assumed the trip would be short and had not prepared. Once at the shop, we spent an obscene amount of money on Cokes as we took into account all of the people we would share with. The canned drinks already ran well over market price due to the remote location. Armed now with heavy, bulging plastic bags we slowly made our way back into the dingy, attempting to balance across the searing hot planks.

Handing a Coke to our kind boat driver, we made our way back to the main building. We then decided to trudge with our goods through the grounds, behind the fish processing plant, to the open air markets.

I never could get used to having eyes follow my every move due to my obvious foreigner status. The people in the markets were exceptionally lethargic in the oppressive afternoon heat. Huge blocks of sago and fried dough lined rows along with sundried fish, crabs, and wilting greens. The smell of raw seafood combined with swarms of flies made me want to cut our visit short. The familiar telltale red stains of betel nut spit covered the packed earth.

We located the garlic and a few other rare food items, paid our *kina*, and headed back to the shade of the station. We found out our vessel had arrived just in time for lunch break, so our driver was at the Chinese shop having tea with the owners. It also meant the new lumber would not even start to be cut until after the break.

I gritted my teeth, "Short trip, indeed."

Justin and Joe graciously offered us their empty air-conditioned office as a place of refuge during our wait.

Bec sprawled out on the floor for a bit, feeling guilty for leaving her son behind. She knew he would be getting hungry and would miss her. I sat in an office chair, propping my feet on the desk. We had not experienced the convenience of air-con in weeks. The blast of frosty air was almost painful to my senses. Hungry and cold, I had every desire to hibernate until it was time to leave.

After the lunch hour passed, we emerged back into the heat to make sure our driver would know where to find us. Hours passed, but we still had no sign of our ride. No one was in any rush to leave. Justin kept us company, missing the companionship of his native Kiwis. Sucking on some coffee candies to stave the hunger, we chatted in the shade.

Baimuru and Kapuna were examples of modern progress in the remote bush. While Kapuna was cheerful, lush, and exuded tropical beauty, Baimuru was grey and dirty. Due to heavy equipment and large machinery driving through, the grass was deeply imbedded with muddy ruts. The stench of fish filled the air. Clouds accumulated overhead as we waited. *Bua* stained the ground around us.

Enormous logs floated just off the sawdust strewn shores. Many of the logs were bound together with crude tents pitched on top of them. Locals would float the timber down the river to Baimuru, living on top of it for the long journeys. There they would sell it to the lumber yard. Many times those earnings were poured back into Baimuru as the locals purchased cigarettes, betel nut, or alcohol from the stores. Coke cans also littered the rivers closest to this station. A cellphone tower sat atop the sawmill with satellite dishes peeking from clapboard huts.

It was one of the sad realities that modern "progress" brings with it.

My heart was saddened in realizing one of the greatest injustices the developed world could bring to a place like the Gulf Province was convincing the people of the area they were poor and needed things they never relied on to live before.

While adequate medical care is a necessity, this was a place filled with people who had an incredible ability to survive harsh jungle conditions, knowing how to live efficiently and well off of the land around them. Gardens thrived.

While materialistically poor, the people of this area are far from being destitute. The family structure was their form of insurance; villagers took care of each other's needs as they arose. Then, development came bringing both the good and the ugly. Modernization came in the form of much needed improvements to the quality of life, but it also brought alcohol, rubbish from packaging, pollution from mines and plants, and a stripping of the land's resources like fish.

I sat, surveying my surroundings and contemplating the depth of this. Could poverty actually be the result of imprudent progress? Was discontent less likely to have existed before we brought in our outside conveniences, instilling the desire for unnecessary items? What did wisdom in community development look like? Where do we draw the line between necessary rights and excessiveness? Was that an outsider's decision to make?

I had come from America where the dream was to stay one materialistic step ahead of the masses. I hated to see the possibility of this beautiful region falling victim of the same elusive fulfillment.

Finally, our canoe arrived and the men loaded the freshly cut timber.

Our return was slow going due to the load. Bec and I continued in pleasant conversation as the clouds broke loose, unleashing an afternoon rain. The cool breeze of our forward movement made us both a bit sleepy, but there was no comfortable way to stretch out.

The brief storm quickly relented. Soon enough, we were inundated with termites. These horrible creatures formed clouds across the river. Completely invasive, they were flying into our ears, eyes, and down our clothing. Bec opened her umbrella. We huddled close underneath it, with our backs to the bow. We could not swipe them off quickly enough. Removing a few just meant more would take their place. This was our ritual for the next half hour.

Everyone else on the boat crouched at the bottom of the canoe with their shirts pulled up around their ears. Our poor driver just had to endure the ride, watching for logs and debris in the water. True to island time, we arrived back at Kapuna about four hours later than we were told we would. My productive day was shot all in the name of some garlic cloves and canned diabetes.

That evening when I went to shower, wings and dead termites dropped from every bit of clothing I removed. Life in the tropics had its benefits, but this was a repulsive side effect of the climate.

It was worth it, however; I had built a friendship with an amazing person. Levi also survived the long day without his mother. One more notch in the refinement of patience with "Island Time."

THE CHANT

Sitting on the steps, breeze rustling through the palms and flowers nearby I heard chanting. Usually the chant ended in a cheer or laughter, sometimes a combination of the two.

I looked over at the school construction site to my left and saw about twenty men atop planks of wood, slanted up onto a tall post. The tall post was sticking a few meters out of the swamp. As they chanted, they jumped, pushing the post further into the murky flood plain waters.

Some of the efforts were rewarded with quick sinking, other times the timber the men were standing on began to crack as significantly more force was being put on the plank than the actual post being driven. With their chants and their rhythm, however long it took, the posts were going to be driven into the ground. It was one of the many techniques used while building in a swamp.

As an outsider, I was in awe of the ingenuity. I sometimes forget these are people who, for thousands of years, have built in flood plains and swamps. We use civil engineers. They are so in tune with their land; it is second nature.

After the posts were driven, the men wrapped them with a dense, black plastic before cementing them into place. The mucky soil mixed with the cement.

It was hard for me to envision a school built atop this field of posts in the swamp. Kapuna's school was started by Barb. Kapuna Hospital has an elementary and middle school, serving the hospital staff families. It combines New Zealand and PNG curriculum to ensure the students are getting a well-rounded education that is culturally appropriate. The main language of the school is English.

Evolving from Barb Calvert's homeschooling, the school has been growing at an exponential rate. As a young married couple, she and Colin had settled into Kapuna Hospital as the administrative staff. Five children later, she was doing what she never dreamed of, teaching. Soon her children's friends were gathered around her home, wanting to learn as well. A facet to running a hospital is providing an environment for staff to raise their families. Hospital staff was not willing to stay if their children could not receive a good education. The local schools were inconsistent and did not have a high quality curriculum. Additionally, many of them lacked any standardization or government follow-up. Sometimes teachers would disappear for months, still collecting their pay but not actually working. Not only did this leave locals frustrated, it meant their children's education fell on the rare few who were trained well enough to teach.

Before she knew it, Barb had a small school running. It expanded a few grade levels, up to eighth grade. Due to increasing demand, however, when I arrived, new buildings were in process. Dr. Valerie's ex-husband, Bryan, is a contractor and builder and helped design the schools. Their son, Caleb, had come with his wife, Rebecca, and their two small children, Neriah and Levi. Bec's friends from New Zealand, Simon and Brooke, also joined for four weeks.

Working tirelessly in the extreme heat, the guys made incredible progress while there. The local lumber from Baimuru station was some of the most beautiful I had seen.

Months after I left Kapuna, I was in for a pleasant surprise as I flipped through photos of the school dedication and opening. The two buildings were stunning. With so much additional space and colorful murals, all they needed now was some more school staff and the area would be well equipped to continue its expansion of education.

Caleb has also taught all over the world and just finished his degree in administration. He shared his dream to possibly return to Kapuna one day and put together a teacher's training school in the area.

WANTOK AND DINNER

Stools, a rocking chair, a long bench, and random chairs were packed around the faded wooden table. Aesthetically, it was far from a beautiful table, but it was the gathering place for the Calvert family. Kids had done homework there, Uncle Ted had his work spread across it, and games were played around the table. As we all found a place, shuffling elbows and mismatched dishes, this table held some of my fondest memories in Kapuna.

At least a few nights a week, the sun would start to set and the generator would kick on. This signified it was time to hurry across Kapuna to Colin and Barb's house. Upon entering, a scruffy orange cat named Kinzer greeted me. The kitchen, with an old wood burning stove, would be a hive of activity. Most of us would join the final preparations in the kitchen: slicing pineapples, cooking sago, gutting fish, or washing up prep dishes. Others would filter in. Once dinner was ready, Dr. Valerie returned from her run around the pineapple patch, and Grandma had arrived from her house, we held hands in a circle and sang one of their New Zealand benedictions.

Around this table, I became *wantok*, which is family in Papua New Guinea. You do not have to be blood to be *wantok*; you just share the same heart. This concept is similar to other Pacific Island cultures, including Hawaii's Ohana and New Zealand's Whanau. It means we are bound together in community and called to cooperate and honor one another. Having tribal backgrounds, a group of people have a responsibility to defend and take care of the unit. Unlike our celebrated independent thinking in the Western world, wantok takes the whole "tribe" into consideration when making decisions or caring for people. From the minute I had arrived in this bush and Auntie Barb had placed a flower necklace around my neck, I had felt completely loved and accepted by the Kapuna *wantok*.

Some evenings we debated and discussed, solving the world's problems in our tiny corner of the earth. Some evenings we played games like Mafia, most evenings we told and heard stories, and every evening we laughed together. If dining tables were valued by the love and lessons shared around them, Colin and Barb's would be worth a fortune.

THE REAL CROCODILE HUNT

The river was so still, the world was reflected almost perfectly upside down. Other than the occasional noise from a gigantic bat, also known as a flying fox, swooping overhead, our outboard motor was the only noise to break the silence and stillness of the night.

The villages were asleep, but we stalked the predator crocodile.

We would cut the engine at the sight of a croc and glide across the tributary. It was in stark contrast to earlier that evening.

The rain had fallen relentlessly. My heart sank as I ate dinner on my deck, looking out over the bleak fading sun and landscape. The plan was to go on a crocodile hunt that night. While rain made it much more likely to find crocodiles, it made the experience less pleasant for the hunters. I sent up a prayer. I had been looking forward to this quest since our last outing finding fireflies.

I have always had the tendency to look forward to things so much, I crash and burn in disappointment when it does not work out. I also reveled in adventure and time with "the guys." In my ignorance, I felt fearless of the possible consequences of a late night crocodile hunt. Sure, they were mighty predators, but we would be smart, equipped, and in a large dinghy.

AJ and I sat up talking for a while, but she retired to bed around 10 p.m. because she had charge of the church service in the morning and needed to be alert. Gerald, Simon, and Brooke passed the house in the dark, damp outskirts of our garden. Pausing from their spot on the intersecting sidewalk, they shouted up to me.

"We're waiting to see if the rain relents! We'll let you know if we are going."

My patience was wearing thin as the minutes passed. I washed dishes, wiped the counters, and tried not to give in to exhaustion while waiting. Voices and torch light passed my house on its way to the guys' dwelling. I ran to the edge of the deck and saw it was Isaka and Barty.

"Hey, guys, are we going?"

"Pretty sure. We're going to let them know Caleb and Morea are headed over. We will come back and get you before we go."

Island time stressed me out at times. The hands of the clock ticked away after they left. The rain had let up a bit. It would periodically dump torrents and then dissipate again. I had to stop checking the clock. Finally, I saw Caleb's tall shadow crossing to the dark path. I shouted down again. He informed me the hunt was on, but we were going to have coffee first to wake up.

"Bring a cup, the guys do not have enough," he added. I laughed; dishes were limited and frequently went walk-about, never to return.

I ran to grab my things and a coffee mug. My heart raced in expectation. This was going to be a good night. Sprinting over to the dubbed "man cave," I popped my head in to see Gerald heating a kettle while Simon and Brooke lounged shirtless. Caleb had sent Barty off to get Morea and gather the gear.

Once we were all assembled, I hoped we would go. No one else seemed in a rush, however. I had to be reminded the tide was something to be considered when casting off. A large harpoon sat next to me on the floor. Our pile of gear included rain coats, headlamps, a spotlight, petrol, heavy wooden oars, and Bec's homemade snacks.

Coffee was passed around while Morea and Caleb shared both hilarious and chilling tales of previous crocodile expeditions.

We sipped our coffee and laughed as Caleb related the time he and Bec stalked a crocodile for what felt like an eternity. Its red eyes glowed as they approached slowly. The mighty beast stared them down, completely unafraid and unflinching. Finally, getting close enough to throw the harpoon, it struck them that they had been stalking rubbish. The glowing red eyes were just the reflection of a Coke can floating in the river. It is one of the negative signs of the modern world meeting the stone-age.

I looked over at Brooke as his eyes drooped. His curly head pressed against the wall. The guys had spent the entire day building the new school in the immense heat and humidity. I pitied him but hoped he would wake up enough to enjoy the undertaking tonight.

After our coffee was drained, we made one last toilet stop, grabbed the gear, and headed out into the night. Clouds still threatened to unload on us but the rain abated for the moment. Trying to be silent, we followed the sidewalks across the creek to the male students' dorm. We had to cross the narrow pathway that ran through their home to get to the dock where the dinghies were tied up. Passing our supplies down, we climbed through one dinghy and into the furthest one. I was one of the first in and the boat pitched to one side as I stepped, almost dropping a hooked metal bar. Regaining my balance, I helped position everything for the ride. We untied, floating to the jetty where Gerald and Morea jumped on with the rest of the gear.

It was a rough start. Electronics and engine parts were hard to come by in the bush, so sometimes loose wiring made for questionable electrical connections. After wrestling some of the wires, we had the motor going and the spotlight working. Taking off into the night, we quickly made our way across the Wame River looking for muddy banks. I had been sitting on the edge but Gerald motioned for me to sit next to him on the bench seat. Morea navigated, knowing these rivers like we know our neighborhood streets. It was something that always amazed me about PNG. Despite lines of palms and muddy rivers, the locals could tell where they were and the unique traits of the dense foliage. What became more surprising was after a few months in the area, I began to recognize routes. At night, however, it was a different story.

When we first made our way, the clouds still hung heavily overhead. Other than the spotlight and the gathering fireflies, it was dark, very dark.

Caleb was an expert, however, and it did not take long to spot a few small crocodiles in a tributary. Morea silenced the engine; all of us stopped our conversation and waited breathlessly. Brooke sat at the head of the boat, silently gripping the harpoon as we crept up on the glowing red eyes. I could hardly see the creature. All of a sudden, he thrust the harpoon into the water. In a split second, the crocodile disappeared.

This process was repeated over the next hour or so. Sometimes I chatted quietly with Gerald or Morea. Many times, I just stared in awe and wonder at the expanses of stars and galaxies above me with the glowing pulse of fireflies in the trees. I was in the jungle! I imagined what the first explorers to this region must have felt like. How did they carve out a life for themselves from these dense shores?

While Simon sat on the bow with harpoon in hand, he was able to beach a large crocodile. The dinghy ran up onto the muddy banks, the crocodile was in a panic as the spotlight followed it trying to escape us. Before I could take in all that was going on, Barty leapt from the boat into a low hanging branch over the muddy bank, holding a spear, ready to thrust it into the leathery giant. I feared for his life, as he nimbly moved from branch to branch just a few feet over the crocodile. All of this happened with a few seconds, the harpoon was thrown, missing, the meter-long creature escaped and slid back into the waters.

Reality set in. When it was my turn, I was excited but realized if I actually speared a crocodile then what would I do?

The beautiful, breathless, starry night changed again. Here it was about 3 a.m., and I sat scanning the murky waters for red eyes. Gripping the harpoon with purpose, the rain started to come down again. I had brought a slicker but the warm evening and adventure of the night made me feel it would be inappropriate to protect myself from the elements. I wanted the full jungle experience. Drenched, I finally surrendered my position as the crocodile hunter after I became stiff from gripping the front of the dinghy.

It was almost morning when we made it back to Kapuna's jetty with no spoils from the hunt. The tide had receded. At the opening, we had to jump out and push the vessel the hundred yards back to the dock. Caleb told me I could stay in the boat, but Brooke chimed in, "If you don't get out and help, I will throw you in the mud." Fair enough. Since he was the quiet, "nice one," I believed him and scrambled out.

The guys had stripped down to shorts or their underwear. I just hiked up my pants as best as I could. We sank in to our thighs as we pushed. I watched mudfish wiggle into their holes as I shuddered. I hate fish! Each step made me panic I would step on one. The tall reeds towered above my head.

Wet, muddy, exhausted, and with adrenaline coursing through our veins, we survived our crocodile hunt. Unfortunately, so had the crocodiles. No meat for a feast, but one of my favorite memories. A true Land of the Unexpected experience.

BUSH TOILETS

There is no doubt the Calvert family has generations invested in the area. Each one in this talented family uses their own unique gifts to bring something to the Kapuna area. Jadon Calvert, Barb and Colin's son, is currently on that path.

I am going to paraphrase Jadon because he brilliantly summed up community development. In order to see progress with any group of people, you have to find out what drives that people group, what makes them tick. Long-term solutions are not easily found and take a lot of trial and error. It also requires finding leaders and innovators within the community to take on the project as their own. It is their voice that will drive the community to make a project their own and leverage change.

When I interviewed Jadon about his composting toilet project in the Gulf Province, he said, "You do what you can but you cannot push change on people. It has to be something the people want. The community needs to take it on as their own. It cannot be your own agenda."

Often the mistake is made to believe "our ways" are superior. Westerners forget the people of the bush have been farming and surviving in this landscape for thousands of years. Their insight is an absolutely vital contribution to their development.

He shared that outsiders, companies, and missionaries need to check their own agendas before doing a project. If it is to elevate and make them feel good, then it will likely fail. If in their hearts they want to come alongside a community and understand what drives their culture, then they can leverage change. Jadon said his toilet project was received well in Maipia village because he found a local man who was a forward thinker. The man was known for building and creating new things, fixing old things or making them better. He had a strong voice in the community and was already making attempts to create something similar.

Jadon followed his older sisters' footsteps and moved to New Zealand when he was thirteen to finish his education. Living with Uncle Ted's family, he went to high school. He has always loved art and his teachers supported his talent. He said his parents were very encouraging as well. Colin had left school early, discouraged because he pursued what he believed people wanted him to do rather than what he loved doing. Learning from that, he wanted his children to pursue what they loved. Art led to design and Jadon was offered scholarships to university in design. First, he looked at costume design, but a speaker shared about industrial design. Intrigued, Jadon liked the idea of influence and the anthropological side of understanding the human element in design.

At first, he did not necessarily see his degree in industrial design as a way to create positive change in the third world. But, his childhood in Kapuna influenced this area of his life. Jadon grew up seeing companies and missionaries come into the area. He said throughout his childhood he witnessed so many projects fail or hurt a community in the long-term.

I asked what made him take on composting toilets as a project.

In December 2011, Jadon and a university friend traveled to Kapuna on holiday. While they were there, the surrounding area had a huge outbreak of cholera. He knew the hygienic practices of the area were to blame for this outbreak. It resulted in at least 500 deaths across Papua New Guinea, about fifty of those in the Gulf Province.

A report by the World Health Organization stated (Horwood, P. and Greenhill, A. Cholera in Papua New Guinea and the Importance of Safe Water Sources and Sanitation. *Western Pacific Surveillance and Response Journal*, 2012, 3(1):3-5. doi:10.5365/wpsar.2011.2.4.014):

> The presence of cholera in Papua New Guinea is a timely reminder of the declining standard of service delivery in much of the country, which is exemplified by the poor epidemiological data that were collected during the outbreak and the lack of ongoing active surveillance for cholera cases. The concern now is that cholera will persist in the environment and Papua New Guinea will officially become a cholera-endemic country with periodic outbreaks of variable severity. Access to safe drinking-water and adequate sanitation are widely recognized as the key factors to preventing cholera outbreaks. In Papua New Guinea, only approximately 40% of people have access to a safe water supply and adequate sanitation, one of the lowest rates in the Western Pacific Region.

An ulterior motive beyond the severity of cholera, Jadon laughed and told me he just always hated using village toilets. They were hot, smelly, and difficult to access. Many of the toilets emptied into the swampy areas that with high tides or flood waters would spread the human waste to drinking water and gardens. High water could also make the toilets inaccessible. If people cannot access their toilets, they find other options that usually are not safe. Jadon said he always feared eating a village pig because he knew they likely scrounged under the toilets for food. We both took a moment to gag a little at the thought.

In his fourth year, which was his honors year, he knew he had an opportunity. At no other point in his life would he have a full year to dedicate to the research and building of a project like this, so he took it on as his honors project. The majority of his work was done from New Zealand while communicating with his father and leaders in PNG. He said six to seven months were spent doing research and writing briefs.

Jadon's childhood experience in PNG helped him understand the locals' thought processes and ways to build a healthy community. The challenge was finding the core of what was needed to make a product work in the Gulf context. Other questions that had to be answered included: what parts were available, how affordable is it, is it replicable, what is it doing for the community, is it teaching them skills, and what compromises will need to be made along the way? Jadon's project had to be sustainable for the long-term. Anyone living in a jungle context knows the humidity and heat will quickly break down materials.

The first prototype he called his "Rolls Royce toilet." It was the toilet model that would work under all of the best circumstances. From there, he made changes based on adverse circumstances, needs, and available supplies. For instance, some villages are closer to the coast than others. The toilets on lower ground that flood more need to be developed differently than villages on higher ground. Villages on higher ground struggle with the element of distance to get to the toilet. Is it safe for women to get to the toilet at night?

It is an ever-evolving process. Surveys and feedback over the past few years help with the adaptations. He said the product has to be natural for the locals to use. It does not work to introduce too many new things into their culture and has to fit their daily routine. For instance, his model included a function for hand washing. That way, people would not have to do much additional work for this important hygienic step.

After his research and briefs, Jadon then worked on funding. His prototype used 55 gallon polyethylene drums. These are available through a partnership with the local oil companies. The oil companies have a social responsibility to the region but do not always follow through on obligations without outsiders stepping in.

So far, he has about twelve different toilets, although not one of them completely matches his final design. Each village and builders have put their own ideas and personal touches into it. Papua New Guinea is a hands-on culture. Jadon found men within the community to build so they could explain the functions and purpose to the other men in the village as they worked on it. It helped everyone understand the concepts behind how to build the toilet—understanding by doing.

His goal is much larger scale: to put about 250 toilets into the area. While a few major agencies have expressed interest, he struggles with the lack of funding. Most agencies need to see numbers and results, but long-term sustainability is not measureable over a short period of time. Once again, it is about cultural perspective. A lot of outside organizations think in terms of Western values, whereas, Papua New Guineans value different outcomes. There needs to be a melding of ideals.

I asked if hygienic education was a part of the toilet project. Do the locals understand why it is important? Jadon said it was an element. He worked a lot with Dorothy Omae, Kavila's wife—a local politician—on this end. Not only is she a woman of influence in the area, but women are the population to target with education. The men want to know the logistics of the craftsmanship, while the women want to know how they can protect and strengthen their family's health. Dorothy would teach the women while the men worked on the physical end of the project. The mothers are the people in the home with the most influence on their children's education. If the mother understands the health concepts, then the children will be taught it.

He did note that introducing too many ideas into a project is an element of failure seen in the past. Things need to be addressed one step at a time. For instance, a clean water project done in many of the villages required villages to have a hand washing system set up before they would get their water tanks. Many villages quickly threw together a hand washing station. But, when it was followed up on, they were not maintaining it or changing out the stagnant, dirty water. It completely defeated the purpose. The washing stations took a lot of additional work and were not natural to the locals, therefore, quickly abandoned. Had a project been focused on understanding the local mindset and resources, and educating on the purpose of sanitation, it would have likely been a lot more successful than just a tacked-on requirement.

One measureable success that Jadon found when he traveled to PNG to check his prototypes was that they decreased the amount of flies and mosquitoes the toilets attracted, thus reducing insect-borne disease such as malaria.

Another success was seeing Kila Sam, born with spinal bifida, have access to a composting toilet. He has been a frequent patient to Kapuna Hospital over the years. Since he cannot use his legs, a normal pit toilet is impossible for him to access. Jadon's project provided Kila with an accessible toilet, improving his quality of life greatly. It is one of the benefits of Jadon having such close ties to the community. He can make unique changes to his project based on individual community needs, as opposed to an organization coming in and working based off of a larger scale model.

While it will be a long time before the true success of the project is shown, Unicef has shown an interest and might replicate Jadon's work in places like Fiji. Of course, it will require some evolution based on culture and village needs and resources there.

Jadon's work, however, is just another element of the impact Kapuna Hospital is having on the Gulf Province. The Calvert family is Papua New Guinean at heart. This is their nation and they have taken responsibility for being a part of its positive forward motion. The work has become a family affair. It is proof that reinventing the wheel is not necessary to see positive change.

THE PREGNANCY DILEMMA

A heavy knocking was heard at the door. It was a drizzly and cool Friday night, as drizzly and cool as one can get in a hot, tropical jungle. I was sitting in the "man cave" kitchen talking to Gerald while he experimented with coconut oil.

I jumped up to let in Beth whose voice I recognized on the other side of the door. As the door flung wide open, she wasted no time asking us for our blood types.

"I have no idea what mine is," I stammered. "What's happened? I can let you do a test of mine if you need to."

I hate needles and blood but also knew that if it came to helping someone I could not hesitate to give. Gerald went to search for where he had written down his blood type while Beth waited.

"Do you really want to know?" Dr. Beth asked studying my face, "How squeamish are you?"

"I can take it," I responded fully knowing I do not handle anything medical well but have been learning out of necessity and exposure.

She began to describe the horrific situation the hospital's new patient was in.

The young woman, just fifteen years old, had gone into labor days, if not a week earlier. As the labor carried on and the pains got closer together, it was clear that something was wrong. In her remote bush village, her only option was to find the nearest clinic as quickly as possible. But, it was already much too late.

She made the treacherous journey in a dinghy to the health center at Karati. Upon arrival, the Community Healthcare Worker (CHW) was shocked by the task at hand. This exhausted teen could not deliver this baby. The CHW jumped into action with the skill and knowledge of an experienced woman faced with hard medical challenges and limited resources.

She attempted a ventouse extraction using vacuum suction to help get the baby out with no success.

With death for mother and baby looming, the CHW instructed them to make their way to the hospital. The trip was not an easy one. Their fiberglass dinghy with an outboard motor took about six hours. For most locals, paddling in a canoe would have taken a day or more, but time was against them.

One can only imagine what this young woman went through amidst painful contractions, becoming septic, eclampsic, with the sun beating down on her relentlessly in the boat during the day while the threat of crocodiles and getting lost loomed at night. Did she even have enough to drink or eat during her journey?

By the time she arrived at Kapuna that Friday evening, the baby had long been dead. Stuck in the birth canal, the doctors and nurses did not have many options. The signs of eclampsia were clear. Saving this mother's life was utmost in the medical staff's minds.

The molecular cause of preeclampsia and eclampsia still puzzles doctors. Usual signs are hypertension, edema, and protein in the urine while pregnant; this puts both mother and baby at high risk for seizures and even death. It is an exceptionally unusual occurrence in places like Papua New Guinea, while much more common in the Western world for unknown reasons.

After failed attempts at ventouse extraction, options narrowed. It was either symphisiotomy—a surgery to split a ligament, opening the young woman's pelvis more to remove the baby, or perform the horrific task of disassembling the baby to remove him. The sheen of tears in the doctor's eyes portrayed what I knew; a destructive delivery of the baby was horrendous beyond words. It was an option the Kapuna doctors hate to perform, but they knew the mother was the one they had to save now. They explained the process to the young woman and her family; then, the unpleasant task began.

In the midst of it all, her cervix tore while delivering skull fragments. Severe bleeding began.

At just fifteen with two miscarriages in the past few years, this young woman not only endured the loss of her third child but now her life was hanging in the balance. Unfortunately, her story is not singular for the women of remote Papua New Guinea. Due to many factors, PNG is an area that sees one in seven women die in childbirth.

While many PNG women are now married in their late teens to early twenties, it is not uncommon to find very young brides. The people of the Gulf Province of Papua New Guinea already tend to be slight in bone structure and stature genetically. Pairing the women's small frame with a still immature and developing body puts a huge strain on them if an early pregnancy should occur.

With limited knowledge and limited access to birth control options, getting pregnant is pretty much inevitable for a young bride. Even if the woman has the option of birth control, the men govern these decisions. If they want more children, the husband can veto the use of birth control. Many times Valerie, Beth, and Patrick have been frustrated after numerous conversations with men about the risk to their wives and future children if another pregnancy should occur. It does not mean the man does not care about his wife, it usually means he just wants to build his legacy, especially through sons. Death in remote PNG is also very much a part of daily life, unlike the sacred, feared, sheltered occurrence it can be to people in the Western world. It does not necessarily have the same hold on people there.

With dense jungle and beautiful but harsh terrain making up the landscape of the Gulf Province, the vast river systems provide about the only plausible mode of transportation for this area. The people of the Gulf are extraordinary navigators and mariners in these murky, snaking rivers. But, with nautical resources limited to mostly dugout canoes, carved paddles, and the occasional outboard motor, travel can be arduous even for the best of them. Throw in exposure to rain or an unyielding sun and the harshness multiplies.

To add to the already difficult situations, a lack of prenatal education can leave people in the villages without proper knowledge for tending to pregnant women and related complications. Sometimes cultural or superstitious practices like women having to give birth outside, regardless of weather, will also complicate circumstances.

Finally, the fastest outboard motor will not completely alleviate the lack of medical availability. While Community Healthcare Workers are distributed throughout the Gulf at clinics and stations, their training is limited. The Gulf only boasts three hospitals to care for its vast population. It is not just this area, however.

The highlands are faced with similar issues. Travel is difficult over rough mountain terrain and very few roadways. The wet season renders the steep embankments life threatening. Despite the incredible strength of highlanders, medical emergencies are virtually impossible to address in their remoteness. Organizations like Mission Aviation Fellowship (MAF) and Wycliffe-affiliated Summer Institute of Linguistics (SIL) will send planes and helicopters in to pick up patients. However, not every village is outfitted with communication systems. Plus, night time, constantly changing weather, and poor runway conditions will make it next to impossible for flights to come in or leave. It also means getting the sick person to a station with a radio and an airstrip. So many factors hang in the balance.

I had dinner with a couple of SIL pilots when I was staying in Port Moresby. They shared tales of flights around PNG. Due to landing strips not having lighting, they have to do their work within limited daylight hours. There is also a limited number of fueling stations and weather can make landing strips impossible to land on at times. It has stranded them in many situations, sometimes for days with heavy fog coverage. One time, their plane was about to take off, got stuck in the mud, and almost flipped face down as the propeller trimmed the grass on the airstrip.

Our own flight in to Port Moresby was proof of their incredible skill and the tough task they have. Our clear and smooth flight changed in a matter of minutes as we flew directly into a thunderstorm. For the next hour, we were completely blind in the dense, gray clouds. Bouncing all over the sky, they relied solely on their instruments. We did not have any visual references at all until we were almost on the Port Moresby tarmac.

VICTORY AND LOSS

If transportation is not a massive risk to mothers in labor, then knowledge can be. High risk pregnancies are not necessarily recognized in time due to the lack of access to prenatal clinics, so preventative treatment is not sought and the mother may not know there is a problem. Many times, medical victories mean making the best out of a seemingly hopeless situation. Sometimes even with lives being saved, there is pain and loss. (Names in this story have been changed to protect privacy of the patient and people involved.)

Before I arrived in Kapuna, a doctor asked for prayer for one of the patients. Leah* is a school teacher from a coastal region and was pregnant with her first child. Like many women, she arrived at Kapuna Hospital a few weeks before her child was expected, knowing she would be in labor soon. The staff noted a bit of leg swelling but had not run any eclampsia tests, so were unaware to alert the doctor of problems.

As the doctor made her rounds later that day, she was alarmed by Leah's condition. The woman was in severe pre-eclampsic state with every symptom. The local staff does not normally see this condition, as apparently it is very rare in the Gulf Province. Since the doctor was from a Western country, she knew this was life threatening to both mother and baby. The only cure for eclampsia is to give birth, but the process of giving birth elevates the risks.

While writing this book, a high school friend in America, Jeni, died from strokes and seizures due to eclampsia when she gave birth to her son. Despite incredible care and medical advances around the world, this poses an incredible risk for mother and baby. In Kapuna, the doctor knew this and acted quickly to set her up on a regime of medications.

The weight of being only one of two doctors for 30,000 people in the Gulf Province hung heavily in this moment.

It came down to referring Leah to a larger hospital equipped to handle surgery for the expectant mother. Kerema Hospital was their closest option. After getting the local oil company to agree to send their helicopter for the medevac, the doctor attempted to reach Kerema to inform them of Leah and her situation. After many attempts to reach the hospital, she was informed there were no doctors currently at Kerema. A series of bad weather and unfortunate events rendered the hospital doctor-less at the moment.

This incident was not a solitary predicament. As if three hospitals for the province was not already limiting, not having a full, consistent staff at each of them is even more restrictive. After all, doctors do need to take breaks, leave for training and upskilling, or move on to another hospital.

Before the Kapuna staff could make another move, they had to have the consent of the husband. He was in their village far away. Short of sending someone to pick him up, there was no way to get in touch with him for permission to move his wife or operate.

Per most serious medical cases in Kapuna, the staff pray and believe the impossible will be solved. Early the following morning, the doctor awoke and soon was met by the emergency helicopter flying into Kapuna. Everyone in the surrounding area sprinted to the swampy grasses in front of the hospital to meet this unusual sight. With hardly any time to react, the helicopter pilot informed the doctors they were flying straight to Port Moresby.

The staff rounded up necessary emergency supplies, while patient and doctor were loaded. They took off for the capital city. In less than 24 hours, the miracle of answered prayers had occurred, the approval fell into place, and the helicopter unknowingly rerouted their trip to the best destination for Leah.

Hours later, they landed in Port Moresby without incident and were immediately whisked off to the maternity wing of the hospital.

Leah's story does not end there. Due to that incredible miracle, the doctors' quick response, and assistance from the oil company, her life was saved. Unfortunately, the baby had a number of health complications and did not make it. We all hope and pray this beautiful teacher will have a future full of health and even one day, children.

No matter the decision made by a medical professional, life and death can be completely outside of anyone's control. The doctors knew both lives would have been lost had they not moved her to Port Moresby.

WHEN NATURE IS AGAINST US

Dr. Patrick had come for a visit. The minute this young, unassuming Papua New Guinean started to talk I could sense an incredible intelligence and perspective that surpassed his twenty-some years of life. He possessed a fantastic sense of humor, as well. A month later I met his sister, Arabella, and realized it was a family trait. She had the same big smile and brilliant outlook on life.

Born in Papua New Guinea, his parents divorced when he was just a small boy. He and his sister moved to the Land Down Under after his mother married an Australian man when Dr. Patrick was eight or nine years old. Childhood in Australia set him up well educationally and culturally to return to PNG as a young adult.

In 2002, he returned to Port Moresby where he attended the University of Papua New Guinea. He started out with about 400-500 others doing science foundation courses. Through that, the students were narrowed down based on grades and interests. Patrick was one of those chosen to enter the medical school. He joined about 40 others who had been chosen. After his studies, Patrick spent two years doing a medical residency in Port Moresby and Alotau where he did a rotation of specialties.

It was through the residency program that he ended up in Kapuna and Kikori, where he was supposed to spend three months doing a rural placement. It was trial by fire as he finished his one week orientation and was then left to practice as the only doctor on the grounds at Kikori Hospital. He started in December 2012 and his three months stretched into over 14 months. He was waiting for a job, but realized in the midst of it, that he really loved Kikori Hospital and his work there. More than anything, a few minutes into a conversation, I could tell he really loved his patients in Kikori.

When he came to visit Kapuna Hospital, Dr. Patrick was brimming with stories from Kikori where he served as the sole doctor. We sat around the dinner table at Uncle Colin's, packed in tightly, listening to a New Zealand doctor-in-training, Ben, and Dr. Patrick give accounts of life at "the other hospital." With a wide grin, Dr. Patrick began his tale of the day nature was against his patients.

He had four hospital patients in a row, lying in their beds. The first had been bitten on the right arm by a crocodile. It was a miracle he was not killed. The second one had his leg ripped open by a wild pig. The third was a snake bite. Finally, the fourth victim was using an ax to unwittingly chop down a tree possessing a wasps' nest. Soon, the nest dropped and wasps descended on him. As he went to run away with his ax flung over his shoulder, the ax fell, splicing open his calf.

Patrick let out a laugh and we all joined in. "Nature was definitely against us that day!"

Leaning in, we were all intrigued by the crocodile victim and asked him to revisit the story. While the hospitals here have crocodile bite injuries coming in from time to time, we always marvel at the people who manage to escape this mighty predator.

The local man had been on a hunt through the swampy bush with his dogs. As he walked through the tangled growth, his dogs let out a resounding bay and took off after a bandicoot—a large rat-like marsupial that lives in the bush. It makes for a filling and delicious dinner if caught.

He paused, looking for the dogs that were quickly gone from sight. The animals then completely changed direction, switching back, and went racing past him, the terrified bandicoot fleeing for his life. The marsupial then jumped into the swampy river waters nearby. Panicked, the poor creature realized it could not swim and thrashed around.

The man saw this as his opportunity to get his dinner. He entered the water up to his waist and went after the unfortunate bandicoot. He was so focused on his future dinner, the man failed to see a large crocodile waiting just feet away. Just as he was reaching for the bandicoot, the crocodile reached for the man. Chomping down on his right arm up to the shoulder, the crocodile was about to drag him under.

I can only imagine how time must have almost stopped for the crocodile victim. The situation had turned from hunter to hunted almost instantaneously, and the hunting dog instinct took over. The dogs, risking their own lives, jumped in the water and attacked the crocodile who eventually released their master.

With a badly mutilated arm and adrenaline coursing through his veins, the man made his way home. His relatives loaded him into a canoe and took him on the twelve hour ride to Kikori Hospital.

In the darkness of 3 a.m., Dr. Patrick was awakened by two apologetic staff who told him he had a crocodile victim waiting. He said they had significantly downplayed the man's injuries. He was not prepared for what he was about to witness as he left his home in the dead of the night. Groggily, he came in to check the injury. He was horrified at the severely swollen, bruised, and bloodied appendage. There was little he could do until the bleeding and swelling went down.

This is where the victim laid, elevating and compressing the arm, next to his commiserating roommates who also suffered from the harshness of nature. Some would say the man was unfortunate, but surviving a croc attack may actually mean the opposite; he was blessed to be alive.

In the coastal lands of Papua New Guinea, nature is not always man's ally.

THE DEVASTATION OF AIDS

According to reports by the UN, PNG is estimated to have one of the worst HIV/AIDS epidemics in the Asia and Pacific Island Region. Much of this stems from a lack of understanding about the disease and its causes. Remoteness to regions again plays a role in reaching isolated people with this vital information. It is a difficult and time-consuming task, especially when some people groups and villages have yet to be discovered.

When you do finally get to a remote area, extensive education about biology and science would have to be shared before you could expect people to believe in unseen, microscopic viruses.

Another factor is the sexual habits, like polygamy. Then there is the lack of access to preventative medical measures or the diagnosis. Essentially, there is no easy solution and volumes of books could be written on the topic.

After all, we see in many cultures that people who even bear the knowledge do not always act responsibly in their sexual behavior.

Some stories have healing and hope. Most stories carry a bittersweet ending. Regardless of culture or background, many people who have lived for a time on this earth will tell you most of life is far from ideal yet carries sweetness and moments of joy. There are people who do not understand the mingled sweetness, however. Sometimes circumstances just break a heart. Dr. Patrick could hardly sit still when he shared about Helen.

He had been telling me about the social acceptance of domestic violence in the Kikori area. He said, "In some parts of PNG it is frowned upon but here there is a lot. A woman's role is to give birth and raise kids. Women are dispensable. Many men have multiple wives."

I could tell the words were like gall in his mouth. He despised this aspect of his work, tending to battered women only to send them back to the hard life. Patrick was a man who greatly admired his mother and looked upon his sister as a best friend. I could tell that like the many great men I had met across PNG, he did not hold with the belief that women were second-class to men.

With a heavy heart, he began to talk about Helen, who was a happy girl of about fifteen or sixteen. She had been bought by a man of wealth and influence in another village to be his fifth wife. In less than a month after taking Helen as his wife, his illness overtook him and he sought treatment at Kikori Hospital. Dr. Patrick knew after one look that the man was dying of tuberculosis. He was spitting up blood. After a few more tests, the man was also informed he was positive for HIV. Dr. Patrick and staff counseled the man, advising him to take care not to infect the rest of his family.

Unconcerned for his expendable wives, the man went home to die, though not before laying the blame for his illness at Helen's feet, even though she was clearly not the source for the disease. A few days later, the man died. His other wives also blamed young Helen, although he had been sick long before he took her as a wife. The battle grew ugly against her and soon she found herself sick.

Hoping against all odds for a good prognosis, Dr. Patrick tested her for TB and HIV. She was positive for both. Rather than being left to live out her life in peace without a husband, her parents went to battle with the man's family. They, who had sold her to the cruel man in the first place, were seeking to benefit from his death and her illness. Using her disease as a ground for monetary gain, her parents had little regard for her wellness in the midst of the judicial battle. Sweet Helen treated merely as a possession never got a say and likely never reaped any compensation for her difficult life.

Our hope by sharing Helen's story is to spread HIV and AIDS awareness, preventing the spread and devastating effects of the disease. This is the continued work of Kikori and Kapuna Hospitals. Some of it depends on awareness, but some things will not change until the people of the Gulf Province can acknowledge that both men and women hold incredible value.

In December, I was invited to join Kapuna's events for World AIDS Day.

Crowds filled the covered walkways at the front of Kapuna Hospital. Cheers and claps rose heartily as the patients and local residents watched skits, performed to entertain but also to raise awareness on World AIDS Day about the sizable spread of HIV/AIDS around the globe.

Soon after, Dr. Valerie Archer and many of the medical staff took the microphone to share information about HIV/AIDS and its devastating effects on Papua New Guinea. They shared not only statistics within the nation but also preventative measures and healthy living habits that would put a stop to the infection and spread of AIDS.

After the presentation, they put together a game for those in attendance to check their knowledge of the disease.

A march made up of the staff and attendees took them around Kapuna. The march was to raise awareness and have the people stop and think about the spread of HIV in their local communities. Morea and other men spoke up against domestic violence as well.

The afternoon was filled with games and events for the children. The hope was to plant seeds in the youth to see the next generation have a greater understanding of AIDS and practice healthier lifestyles. At the end of the week, a few videos on healthy lifestyle practices were screened by the local residents to further their understanding.

The event was not meant for just Kapuna, however. The staff took dinghies and traveled to many neighboring villages to carry out the task of raising awareness.

World AIDS Day is an important event in the area; life and death in Papua New Guinea hinges on understanding this disease. We hope that one day it will be more prevention than treatment.

DOMESTIC VIOLENCE

The urgent voices called from below, just minutes before the generator was turned off for the evening. My roommate, Dr. Beth, scrambled downstairs to meet with our unexpected guests. As she opened the door, I recognized the two men as familiar medical staff in Kapuna.

"A woman has been stabbed. You need to come," one of them said to Beth.

She grabbed her bag and keys, following them into the night.

Hours later when she returned, I got the full spectrum of what had taken place.

A woman, at the hospital for her antenatal care, got into a domestic dispute with her husband. In the midst of the heated argument, he stabbed her in the chest with a pair of scissors. There was a high possibility of a lung collapse and internal bleeding. Stab wounds are never easy cases, even in a state-of-the-art hospital.

All of this was made more complicated by the lack of diagnostic equipment in Kapuna. Without an x-ray machine, the doctors and nurses have to make educated guesses about the state of the lungs and if there is blood pooling in them. There is significantly more margin for error.

This remote location has its myriad of challenges due to isolation and the fact that it services around 30,000 people. Added to these challenges is the element of unnecessary violence. Outside of tuberculosis and births, a main reason for patients to arrive at the hospital is as a result of this violence—mostly domestic violence.

The next morning, the woman was in stable but still bad condition. With only one more month of pregnancy left, her chest cavity was filled with blood. A chest drain was prepared but thankfully was not needed in the end.

In the midst of treating a panicked, angry woman with a stab wound, the doctors had to face another trial. While treating their patient, the doctors had to convince local men not to retaliate on the abuser. The result would likely be another patient in the bed next to his stabbed wife.

How do you deal with a deeply imbedded culture of violence? Wife bashing and sexual abuse are not always considered very negative sins in this dense jungle area. Not only is it easy to hide, but it's not necessarily looked down upon either. The result is a people who live to expect nothing less.

A circle of violence spirals when people and family retaliate against the abuse. The staff at Kapuna Hospital tries to respond with grace while hoping their own actions will speak volumes. If they had found the escaped abusive husband, they would have doled out consequences, but hoped to do so in a way to teach him a better way to treat his wife.

Brutal treatment from men is not everywhere in PNG. There are exceptions. While domestic violence needs addressing, it would be unjust of me to not give incredible credit to so many who break the cycle of brutality. I have met several in my travels who advocate, love, and defend the opposite sex.

An Australian friend living in Papua New Guinea recently shared the face of a handsome young PNG man on social media. He was a promising Olympian and kickboxer. He died from severe knife wounds while defending his sister from gang assault. Deeply grieved by the senseless loss, the young man deserves the applause of a hero.

THE PETTERSONS

I met Debbie Petterson via email weeks before I went to Kapuna. She was in charge of organizing my flight out to the bush. After a few short paragraphs, I was eager to meet the coffee-loving Kiwi on the other end of the computer. I could already tell she was a kindred spirit with an incredible sense of humor. Upon arrival at Kapuna, I noted that many of the household items I came across were labeled "Petterson."

I had to wait four weeks to meet her in person since, upon my arrival, she and Robbie traveled to the highlands working for Summer Institute of Linguistics (SIL)—a branch of Wycliffe.

I was not disappointed the day she returned three weeks later. She shouted at me from the sidewalk outside my bush house. One of the first comments she made was, "One thing you'll learn about me is I am crazy."

A few minutes later, she produced a slice of chocolate pie for me. She had brought it back on her flight from the Highlands after taking part in an American Thanksgiving celebration.

I knew then I would officially fit in well. Debbie is "crazy" in all the right ways with her big smile and absurd, wonderful sense of humor, as well as her gift for making a home in this remote tropical land. I soon learned Debbie and Robbie were the people to go to if one needed things, especially a smile. Debbie was also remarkably skilled with her power tools and machete.

Debbie is a fun, attention-seeking ball of energy, complimented by Robbie who is mostly calm, thoughtful, quieter, and very knowledgeable. The corners of his mouth constantly twitched into a smirk as he either laughed at his wife's antics or came up with a few quick responses of his own. Their personalities balanced so well. Both are absolutely brilliant people with the gift of adaptability. Of course, Debbie attributes some of that to the hard years they put in at the beginning of their lives in Papua New Guinea.

Back when Robbie was 21, he was friends with a missionary in PNG. The man invited him to visit a small village in the Gulf Province. With a background focus in computers, Robbie also had an interest in languages and literacy. It did not take much for his interest in language work in PNG to flourish.

Robert Graham Petterson married Deborah Anne Edwards on May 9, 1981. A year later, they were in Australia for language, anthropology, and literacy training with SIL. The training helped them better understand and acclimate to the tribal, bush life, while learning the language and creating an alphabet to teach reading and writing.

In 1984, they visited the village of Kopi, just ten miles north of Kikori, for six weeks. With their first born, Timothy, in tow, they moved to an aid post house in Kopi, in November 1984. In that time, they built their own bush home and began work. There was no plumbing, a drop toilet, meals were cooked on a borrowed wood-burning stove, and the family washed in the river. Eventually they saved money and got a small gas stove for their home.

In 1985, the Pettersons were invited to a camp out in the bush. There they met Colin and Barb Calvert, bonding over their native New Zealand heritage and life in the Gulf Province. Not long after, their second son, Jonathan, was born at Kapuna Hospital. Just a few days old, Debbie recalls her incredible nervousness for many hours in their dugout canoe as they brought Jonathan home to Kopi. They were not the proud owners of their fiberglass dinghy yet. Like the locals, when it was time to check out of Kapuna with Jonathan clutched tightly to her chest, Debbie would have stood at Kapuna's jetty. After handing the baby to someone, she would step into the unstable, wooden vessel, setting herself and her hospital bag at the bottom of the canoe. Over four hours, fear of capsizing with a newborn likely nagged in the back of the mother's mind.

Thankfully Jonathan survived the ride and his childhood in the Gulf Province. Their daughter, Miriam, was also born a few years later, completing the Petterson family.

Nine years were spent in Kopi working on their translation project. They finished one third of the New Testament, a song book, and a dictionary in the local dialect.

Additionally, they experienced the negative impacts of progress during that time when an oil company set up a huge operation in the region causing a lot of social disruption. As the surrounding area was being shaken up by the stripping of the land's resources, the Pettersons' financial wells were drying up. Their home church had lost interest during that time and no longer wanted to support them. Heartbroken, the family moved back to New Zealand in 1993. Robbie got a job teaching information systems (computers) and literacy at a local university.

The three Petterson children struggled the most in transitioning back to New Zealand. PNG was the only home they had known. In 1997, Robbie and Debbie were able to return to PNG to do short-term research work, and in 1999 they did the same again with their children, and then in 2002 Robbie got a sabbatical for a longer stay, again with the family. This was proof their hearts were still in the Land of the Unexpected. In 2004 Robbie went back for a brief literacy project sponsored by Kapuna. This was followed by a larger literacy project from 2005 to 2007.

Using their time in New Zealand to reconnect with friends and churches, they raised a lot more financial backing to return long-term in 2007. Back with SIL, their focus had shifted from mainly translation work towards more literacy. Their permanent home was moved to Kapuna, although they stayed in villages frequently running writers' or translation workshops. They have worked with at least eleven language groups for literacy and five language groups for translation. They have also played a role in the translation of the Jesus film for local dialects. Robbie is fluent in a number of local languages and also surprised us by speaking Maori, the tribal language of New Zealand. Since their translations finished recently, they have been doing consultation, reviews, and checks for other translations.

Learning from years of experience, Debbie was the master at setting up a home in the bush. She always had hidden stashes of goodies like cheese and chocolate, vital for a Westerner's long-term survival.

Early on a Saturday morning, I went out onto my deck for a quiet time. Beth had gone to do rounds at the hospital, so I was alone. I heard Debbie down in the garden, weeding and using her machete on various dying plants. The calm was broken by her scream, as a snake showed itself. Hurrying into view, I saw her sweaty form in dirty gardening clothes and gumboots.

"That's it! I am finished gardening for the day!" She threw up her hands as she talked to me.

I invited her up for a cup of coffee. In typical Debbie fashion, she disappeared into her house only to return with a plate of waffles and powdered milk for the coffee. Robbie came over a little later and we enjoyed our breakfast and coffee together. I know she had a system and stashed good baking ingredients, but I always felt mystified by the inaccessible food she supplied and shared.

As much as she loved all of us, Debbie despised the roosters. The chickens would perch in a tree, eye level with their deck. They were either incredibly brave or incredibly stupid animals because many things, including water balloons, were thrown at them from that deck. We were all tempted to kill the roosters. The Pettersons were just people of action, not idle talk.

If she was not calling the roosters names and throwing things at them, she was whistling and cat-calling the volunteers and staff as we passed their home in the evenings. Everything about them made the Pettersons some of my favorite people. I admire their hard work and bonded with their incredible personalities. One could only wish to aspire to be like "Auntie Debbie."

UNISKRIPT

Every morning they rose with the sun, or maybe it was the roosters? Either way, the Pettersons were up early, brewing coffee and preparing for their day. Come rain or shine with literature and teaching resources exploding from bilums and backpacks, they made the 30 minute walk to Ara'ava, Kapuna's closest village neighbor. Robbie and Debbie are pioneers of a new literacy tool called Uniskript.

Uniskript history is best described on the University of the Nations (UofN) website:

> Uniskript can be traced back to 1446 when King Sejoung launched the Korean alphabet, which triggered a literacy revolution in Korea. In 2002, Korean linguist Dr. Kim Cho shared her doctorate discoveries on the ancient alphabet at the UofN, hoping it could be used to benefit people with poor literacy and no access to the Bible.

The goal is to battle the injustice of illiteracy by creating an iconofeatureal script that represents sounds and is unique to each culture. The script is designed to represent recognizable symbols within the cultural context. For instance, the script created for Ara'Ava used shapes like a bow and arrow or the shape of a dugout canoe. Each script also represents the position of the mouth when making a sound. They are created to be attractive to the people learning them and relevant to the sounds made. It is all based on phonics.

Having started translation and literacy work with SIL in the Gulf Province back in 1984, Robbie and Debbie were excited for this new challenge presented to them in February 2013. Four local educators were selected—Roy Harai, Nelson Moio, Anna Larupa and Esther Ukia—teachers from the Urama and Koriki language communities, who came highly recommended. They travelled to Kona, Hawaii that June with Robbie and Debbie. While it was quite the intense time of training for the Pettersons, the four locals were in for the trip of their lives.

Having grown up in the remote Gulf Province, Roy, Nelson, Anna, and Esther hardly ventured outside their villages, let alone across the world. It was an extreme change going from life in thatched huts and long-drop toilets to the bustling western cities in Hawaii. It was their first time flying and leaving their native Papua New Guinea. One can only imagine the fear mingled with enthusiasm as they traveled across the globe. Robbie and Debbie enjoyed the PNG team's excitement but also carried a lot of responsibility watching over the four, who were intrigued by so many little things during this experience.

The trip had a few hiccups early on as the six travelers landed in Honolulu International Airport. Airport security pulled the Pettersons aside for additional screening while waving on the four PNG natives. Robbie and Debbie tried earnestly to explain to security why they needed to keep together as a group. Uncaring, the security could not grasp the magnitude of their request and took them into a room for screening, leaving the Papua New Guineans to fend for themselves. Panicked at losing their charges, the Pettersons impatiently went through the security screening, anxious to find their team again.

In the meantime, the four Gulf Province villagers did not understand what happened to their leaders. Wandering around the massive international airport, in their broken English they asked random people if they knew where "Uncle Robbie" and "Auntie Debbie" had gone.

After being released, Robbie and Debbie had little time to make their gate but needed to find their team. Running around the airport, worriedly searching for the four, they found them wandering around outside the international terminal not knowing what to do next. They quickly escorted them through security and to the correct terminal for the next flight to Kona.

In an article by Robbie Petterson and Tim Scott with SIL, they describe the three weeks at YWAM Kona:

The PNG team learned how to use Uniskript symbols to represent language sounds, and then developed symbols for Koriki and Urama. After testing the symbols by writing words and sentences, they looked at cultural icons, designs and artifacts, and used these to adapt the basic symbols to ones that had a real "Urama" or "Koriki" home-grown feel to them. The Koriki teachers called their Uniskript alphabet "Koriki Ere," which means "(growth-giving) water for the Koriki," while the Urama pair called theirs "Urama Hura," meaning "the seeds (of learning) for the Urama." They also worked on basic Uniskripts for Tok Pisin and Hiri Motu. The team later developed teaching materials and games and stories for reading practice, using computer fonts created especially for them. An important final step was planning teaching materials for bridging to the Roman alphabet and to help children learning to read English.

After returning to Kapuna, the Pettersons and their team took time to train more of the local educators. If the teachers are not trained correctly, it can result in bad habits being taught and passed down. This makes the work much harder in the long-run when all of those habits have to be broken and relearned by students.

It can take six months to get a child literate in their own language. With Uniskript, it can take a matter of weeks, possibly months. Once a person is trained in Uniskript, learning to read their own language and even English becomes easier due to understanding the theory behind reading and writing.

Ara'ava is a remote, insignificant blip on most of the world's maps, yet this innovative literacy tool was put to the test with over 120 students from three villages.

Similar to Jadon's toilet development, a key to developing literacy in a region is getting the community behind the work. In the past, so often, well-meaning outsiders would bring their ideas and plans for development but not have the backing of the local community. It is presumptuous and a bit arrogant to assume people need or want the change we bring. The Pettersons understood this. They were also such a part of the local fabric; they were *wantok.* They met with village leaders before the project started to ensure it was something the community even wanted. The people in the Purari River area are not used to being the first in innovations. In fact, many are used to feeling left behind by the modern world, so when Robbie and Debbie presented them with the opportunity to be at the head of a new literacy program, they jumped. The village leaders and families were excited for their children to gain this experience.

The Pettersons, along with Hanna Schultz and Melanie Leclerc from SIL, worked with the local teachers to educate the children. Robbie and Debbie believed the best way to train the teachers was to put theory into practice by using Ara'Ava classrooms as the main training grounds. The SIL workers were present to help guide the local teachers, and then debriefed them about what went well and not so well at the end of each day.

The other practice they found effective was to have the children teach it back to the staff. It helped the educators ensure the kids understood the material.

This is the stage they were in when I met the Pettersons. Hanna and Melanie had joined them for five weeks from other locations in Papua New Guinea to be assistants in the process. Over the Christmas holiday break, the students from Ara'ava, Kairimai, and Kai'aravi came each weekday for class. Some traveled via dugout for an hour.

I had very little understanding of Uniskript when I first made my trek to Ara'ava. Little did I know, I would bear witness to the laying of foundational stones for a likely historic game-changer in worldwide literacy.

Per the usual December day, it was already muggy by the time I left at about 9 a.m. A well-worn path meandered past the hospital kitchens, running behind Kapuna. It had poured the previous evening, so the path was slick with mud and ankle deep with water at some points. Stepping off the path and onto the grass to keep my footing, I wandered through banana plantations and other gardens planted by the locals. From time to time, I would pass a group wielding machetes on their way to work their patch of land. At least ten times on the half-hour walk, my balance was tested as I stepped onto a slick log or crude bridge that covered creeks and drains leading to the Wame River. At one point, the path was so flooded I strategized on how to get around. Making my best attempt at a running leap, I hurtled through the air only to miss my mark by a foot. Landing amidst the puddle, I drenched myself from the waist down. The locals walking behind me giggled and said the usual, "Sorry, sorry."

Sorry in PNG is less an apology and more said as a word of sympathy, implying: "We're sorry that happened to you."

Finally making it to the outskirts of Ara'ava, I passed a group of men hollowing out an unfinished canoe. It would hold about twenty people comfortably when complete. The path left the river banks and crops, leading through the middle of homes and yards. Men and women stopped their daily life to smile and wave, calling out greetings as I passed through. The school was on the far end of this long village. As the path opened to a clearing, I spotted the school buildings situated behind the covered village meeting spot.

To my delight, bright eyes followed every movement of the teacher's hands on the chalk boards. The crowded room was full of curly heads, sitting on the floor, and eager hands shooting in the air to answer questions. With the leaders and the families in the community supporting them, students attended very regularly. This helped not only with the advancement of the students but to gauge the success of the program. The first few days were spent testing each child to see which class level they would fall into. The youngest pupil was just four years old. Despite the age cut off at five, Dorine insisted on attending. No one had the heart to turn away a small child from learning.

While it went well for the most part, things were not always smooth. One day Hanna, Melanie, Robbie, and Debbie returned to Kapuna much earlier than usual. Alarmed, I asked what had happened. They informed me an "incident" had occurred at the school. We just had to pray it would blow over enough throughout the community for the program to continue.

While playing a game in class, the students were racing back and forth across the room as sounds were shouted out. One particularly unruly boy was growing more and more excited. In a rambunctious state, he raced across the room, crashing through the thin, woven palm walls. Since the school sat up one story high on stilts, the fall was not a small one. To make matters worse, he happened to fall in the exact spot a giant hole had been dug. He crashed head first into the deep hole, thankfully softened by recent rain.

After they took him to Kapuna Hospital for a check-up, the boy was fine. Thankfully, the fall just shook him up. However, it gave his father cause to become violent against other villagers with whom he had previous problems. Looking for an excuse to stir up trouble, the man started a few fights over the incident, accusing people of poor maintenance to the school building.

Our prayers were answered, however, and by the next day the hole in the wall was patched, and no one was harmed in the excitement. The only difference was the rowdy pupil never returned to class.

After everything calmed, we sighed a breath of relief and laughed that the school had its first "drop-out." Once again, I was reminded that PNG truly is the Land of the Unexpected. Never in my experience had I seen, or would I expect, a child to literally drop from a school building into a hole while playing educational games.

Each morning, the four classrooms buzzed with energy. The village children were riveted on the teachers with eager faces. Hands would shoot up as a teacher asked for volunteers. They followed each move of sounds and symbols. Small clusters of children would group around a pile of cards with the Uniskript symbols. Teachers demonstrated a sound and the kids scrambled to grab the correlating symbol.

I watched as small amounts of water were poured onto the wooden floors. The students dipped their fingers in the water and practiced writing their symbols over and over again on the ground. Bent intently over their work, most hardly noticed me as I stepped among them taking photos with my camera. In the classrooms with the older pupils, I watched as they demonstrated their understanding to their peers through exercises written on the chalkboards. It was clear within a week's time, the students comprehended and excelled at Uniskript.

The school day wrapped up just before noon, after which the teachers and SIL staff would gather for discussion. The Pettersons would get the trainers to break down their work: what went well and what needed improvement. It was a teaching moment for the educators, as this debrief time helped them evaluate their own skills. It was also a time of encouragement, involving much laughter. Like most gatherings in PNG, debrief was more about relationship than anything else.

Returning home for lunch if the tide was high, we heard the tell-tale splash of Robbie and Debbie jumping in the creek to cool off. After a quick swim, they spent their afternoons and evenings doing a lot of behind-the-scenes work. They created books for teaching, written in both Uniskript and the local languages. Pictures had to be included as well. Some were rough sketches, others were clip art. The problem was there was not much clip art to match with culturally relevant sentences.

On one of a few evenings with Julien and Gerald sitting on my deck, Debbie's head popped out of their window. She invited us to come join in the book binding party.

By the dim light of the generator power, we stacked, folded, and stapled together hundreds of books after Robbie spent his afternoon formatting and printing.

Just before a short break for Christmas and New Year's, the Uniskript team gave out the books. It was such a special occasion for the village children. Lined up in rows by class level, they stood outside, waiting their turn to receive the precious gift. Grinning from ear to ear, I snapped photos of the little ones holding their treasure. The teachers implored the children to take good care of books and bring them back to class after the holiday. Almost every child returned daily with the books in hand. Some had even colored in the pictures. Most, if not all, of the villages in the Gulf Province are places where children sharpened pencils with razor blades and many classroom supplies were shared by multiple children. Owning a book is a privilege. Once class resumed, it was clear the students were keen to finish what they had started.

The day before holiday, Robbie and Debbie had driven their dinghy to Ara'ava to transport the books. We willingly jumped in the boat to ride back to Kapuna after wrapping up debrief. The cool breeze off the water was refreshing in the hot afternoon. Debbie volunteered to drive. To our delight, she whipped a few donuts on the Wame in front of the village before we shot up the river to Kapuna.

The tide was going out and we had made it just in time for the canal that runs up to their house to be about half full. It meant we could dock closer, rather than at the jetty. Getting there required maneuvering past tree stumps and debris on the bottom of the narrow waterway. We also had to go under a few small bridges. The motor had to be lifted from the water and the paddles used.

We drifted under the first bridge as Debbie removed the outboard from the water. Seconds later, we heard a splash as Debbie tumbled head first off the back of the boat. Hanna, Melanie, Robbie, and I burst into laughter, along with all the old men sitting along the bridge. We all assumed it was Debbie being funny. Seconds later as she emerged from the water, we realized it was no joke. Pushing off from under the bridge, she had forgotten to let go of the bridge, and then she lost her balance and fell in. Robbie scrambled to help her out. Sopping wet, she scowled at us as we tried to suppress our giggles. I had to break eye contact. The corner of her mouth turned up, telling us her sense of humor was still intact. We quickly apologized and explained we thought she had done it on purpose. I almost felt guilty that it was even funnier because it was an accident. Of course, in the Land of the Unexpected, falling overboard is a risk of the daily commute.

DUGOUT CANOES AND A VILLAGE GOODBYE

Melanie and Hanna had to wrap up the program and leave before graduation. The classroom training of Uniskript had ended in mid-January. On their final day in Ara'Ava, a procession of people filed back to Kapuna with arms laden in gifts. The SIL women were given loads of pineapples, head dresses, shell necklaces, coconuts, and hand-carved spoons, as a token of the parents' gratitude for their work. They worked hard to pack all of the belongings for their flight.

The weekend before they left, the team was invited to Kai'aravi for another goodbye ceremony. Rising early, Melanie and I sat at the end of the jetty awaiting our dugout canoe to transport us. The local teachers had insisted Melanie and Hanna ride with them in the enormous dugout canoe rather than in Robbie and Debbie's dinghy. Hanna had walked to Ara'ava to meet the teachers.

The tide was high while we sat in the morning sun, feet dangling off the edge of the jetty. Slathering on sunscreen for the long ride, we watched the canoe appear in the distance. It could hold between 30-50 people, although at the time, it only had about ten inside. Nervously, we looked at each other and back at the hollowed-out floating tree. The fear in tipping was less about drowning and more about the giant crocodiles that infested the local waters. They pulled up next to the jetty. Hanna was already situated inside with her broad sunhat on.

I had to giggle when I saw her. She reminded me of a British garden party in her flower print meri blouse and sunhat. She sat as regally in the canoe as she would have at a table spread with afternoon tea. She was such a mix of feminine grace and tough, Australian stock. Hanna could sail oceans in ships, work farms on the Italian country side, live in the highlands of Papua New Guinea, all the while sporting an intricately braided hairdo and floral dress. She could sew beautiful crafts, enjoy culture and art, and do it all with a delicate and sweet air about her. She was only one year my senior, yet I held her in such awe that I looked to her for advice and wisdom.

Once the canoe was stabilized along the jetty, I crawled in first. Crouching down, I gripped the sides of the canoe and slowly—very slowly—walked to the middle near Hanna. The men laughed at my clumsiness, as every dip of the vessel made me jump. While it was incredibly long, the canoe was not very wide. My knees knocked on either side while sitting cross-legged. Melanie followed in similar fashion.

The outboard dropped into the water and we jetted off down the river. The first ten minutes were tense. Hanna kept telling me to loosen up but each twist and turn made me rigid with fear that we would tip. I clung to my camera bag, praying we would not go overboard. The locals stood, squatted, and moved nimbly about the boat. I barely breathed. At each bend in the river, the canoe swung wide to take the turns.

Loaded with more people, the Pettersons' dinghy could keep pace with us. After a bit, our bodies adjusted to the motion of the canoe and we chatted freely.

Kai'aravi is significantly smaller than Ara'ava. The banks were decorated with a profusion of flowers and ropes of long grasses. Our canoe pulled alongside the steep banks. We were each helped out and draped with flower necklaces. My fear of tumbling out of the canoe and onto the bank was averted. The exit from the canoe was remarkably fluid.

After briefly hugging and shaking hands, we were ushered into the small church building, already packed with students and their families. Edging our way to the front, we sat on benches facing everyone else. Many speeches were given as leaders, elders, and the local school teacher shared the impact this program had on their children. Then, the Pettersons, Hanna, and Melanie spoke in turn. Gifts were presented, followed by a meal contributed by most of the village families.

Melanie had never tried *Kikirapu* and surveyed the cooked grubs with interest. The locals urged her to try their favorite dish. I warned her as best I could, but Debbie insisted the sago grubs tasted like bacon. I was unsure of what bacon in New Zealand tasted like, but was sure *kikirapu* was nothing like bacon.

Tasting one, she thought it was rather good. The locals then proceeded to heap her plate full of the cooked sago grubs. I cringed inwardly. Minutes later, I looked over and could tell the delicacy did not taste as good as she chewed her way through many. The realization she was eating giant maggots had set in. I returned my attention to my grub-free plate, thankful it was not me eating the maggots.

After lunch, we toured the village with children hanging off our arms and following our steps. I even met six-year-old triplets, a very unusual sight in Papua New Guinea due to birth complications.

We loaded into the dinghy to head home, as the dugout transported children and people back to neighboring villages. I had the chance to experience a seafaring phenomenon: whirlpools. The sands at the bottom of the rivers would shift as the river tide went out, the ocean tide rose, and tributaries met. Opposing currents create whirlpools throughout the river, that, although not particularly strong, if a small boat got caught in one, it could be whipped around and possibly tipped. Robbie skillfully dodged a number of whirlpools as we made our way home that day.

While it is still very much in the beginning stages, the graduation at the end of January 2014 was significant proof for the success of Uniskript. Student after student rose from their seats to clearly and fluently read out Uniskript in their local language. Shy, quiet pupils blossomed with confidence. Even the youngest students had picked up the concept quickly.

Village leaders and parents rose to share their gratitude for the program. They beamed with pride as their children read. Linking the symbols with sounds, their young minds are significantly better equipped for literacy in both their native language and English. Literacy opens their world for expanding education and opportunities. There was also pride in knowing the Gulf Province was at the forefront of the world for this new literacy tool.

THE GERMAN WITH AN ISLANDER'S HEART

"What is one of your favorite things about life in PNG?" I asked with my pen poised to capture his every word.

His dark eyes lit up in jest. "Other than the leeches?" he laughed.

I laughed too. I found it completely unnecessary to take note of Gerald's leech experience. I had heard enough about it to never forget. On one of his first days living in Kapuna, a jungle trek left four leeches attached to his legs. Rather than be repelled by the blood sucking creatures, he was proud. It was part of his initiation to jungle living, a moment signifying he was a real bushman. After all, no one else had as many leeches attached to their legs.

It seemed engrained in his nature to make the most out of every situation. As I sat across from him on my deck in Kapuna, I wondered how much I would have missed if I had never really gotten to know him.

We had both served with Youth with a Mission Medical Ships-Australia (YWAM MSA). Located in Townsville, Queensland, he had literally come to Australia with our ship - the M/V Pacific Link - in 2010 when YWAM Marine Reach in Tauranga, New Zealand donated the ship to Australia. Soon after his move to Australia, this ship engineer and IT guy, traveled to PNG with the medical ship. Through the medical ship, he met the staff at Kapuna Hospital and one of his best friends, Morea. Morea is a PNG hospital staff who is also capable with computers, engine repairs, and just about any skill that might come in handy at Kapuna. Both of them possess the gift of always wanting to know more.

While Gerald previously served in Fiji, there was a moment where he looked at a village shoreline and thought, "What if I just jumped overboard and went and lived there?"

Since then, he desired to not just to travel from village to village but to go live in one. After his commitment with YWAM ended, that is exactly what he had done. Arriving in Kapuna a month prior to me, Gerald was living out his dream. He served in capacities from engine repair, to helping with building the school, to IT work. Jokingly, we referred to him as a "Swiss Army Knife German."

When Kapuna needed special skin graft stretching tools for a burn patient, Gerald invented some. When Caleb and the builders left, Gerald oversaw the finishing of the school, despite having very little construction training. When I desired to rebuild and design Kapuna's old website, Gerald was able to handle all of the background coding for me.

In his free-time, he helped record and produce local songs with Morea, teaching himself piano and guitar.

He is a well-equipped and versatile person. Perfect for this patch of bush and contributing to its development. On top of it all, Gerald was very relational, getting to know many of the locals, spending free time chatting on decks or talking about culture and theology. He appreciated and accepted life at the Island pace, being one of the few German friends of mine with little regard to being on time.

BEACH DAY

Stifling heat had filled December. Many times I visited our freezer to place an ice pack on my neck to cool off.

It was time for another adventure.

Early one Saturday morning, over thirty students, staff, and volunteers lugged supplies to the jetty, waiting to load the aluminum canoe. From person to person, plastic bags with pots, pans, water, and food were passed down the walkway. Finally climbing aboard, I found a place with Dr. Beth, Melanie, and four female students at the front of the canoe.

The canoe was so full, people sat on the platforms connecting the outriggers to the body of the canoe. Our travel was slow due to the weight, but no one seemed to care.

Clouds threatened to rain on our day, but we refused to let them deter us. As we waited, Beth sprayed a glob of sunscreen onto my back. I stubbornly complained I did not need sunscreen. In her greater wisdom, she lectured me on the effects of the tropical sun. It would have been prudent to heed her advice. Later that day, I would wish I had listened as my painfully burned skin made the next few days unpleasant.

Sitting at the nose of the canoe, I enjoyed the spray of water and emerging sunlight as we skillfully navigated tributaries, eventually bringing us to a broad river and the ocean. I listened to Melanie converse in Tok Pisin with the students, trying to discern their conversation.

I was a bit disappointed as we arrived at a slender sandbar covered in driftwood and creeping vines. It was absolutely not what I had pictured for the beach.

The tide was high and as it receded, I could see the merits of the area better. Wielding machetes, the men set to work early to build a shelter. Skillfully cutting large palm leaves, they jumped in the chest deep water and swam them across the chasm between the jungle and the beach. Previously, they had found large branches for structural tresses and wall beams. Enthralled, I watched as the construction came together almost flawlessly. The palms made up the roof, three walls, and flooring. It was a splendid shade.

I decided then and there if I were ever to be stranded on a deserted island, I would choose the company of coastal Papua New Guineans to anyone else.

Sekpain and her friends built a fire, breaking out pots and pans, they were soon filled with boiling oil and *kaukau* slices. As fish and crabs were caught, they were gutted and cooking on fires that cropped up throughout the beach.

We swam, we ran through the sand, we played ball games. Life in Papua New Guinea seemed to bring delight after delight. Friendships blossomed that day.

One of my highlights was going for a walk with Melanie. I was in awe of the young Canadian woman who had left her life behind in Quebec to move to PNG to work in linguistics. We sat on a large bit of drift wood after strolling for a bit. As we shared about life, we spent time in conversation and prayer.

Extreme change of culture and lifestyle can leave one in awed wonder but it can also bring out the worst in personalities as people struggle with loneliness, adjustment, and comparison. Sometimes coworkers can be idolized because we only see their triumphs or the fruit of their labor. It was good for both of us to find out the other person struggled with imperfection. Often times we are our own greatest critics.

Our time of prayer ended with us asking God to confirm His promises to us. Little did we know how that would take shape later in the day.

One of the risks in any swimming of these waters was the crocodile. We were close enough to the ocean to encounter saltwater crocodiles. While it nagged a bit in the back of my mind, I ignored the nagging and enjoyed the cool waters in the heat of the day.

As we prepared to leave and the sun began to lower, the female students and I jumped in one last time, splashing and laughing. Then, to our horror, Sekpain let out a terrified shriek, grabbing at her leg and falling down in the water. Instincts kicked in as we rushed from the water. It felt like an eternity as the worst case scenarios ran through my head. I was unsure of how to respond to a crocodile other than running.

Merely seconds later, Sekpain burst into peals of laughter, teasing us for our horrified response. Adrenaline and heart rate lowering, my brain comprehended that she had faked a crocodile attack. At this point, I turned and ran at her full speed, knocking her back in the water. Splashing her, I scolded her for scaring the daylights out of us.

She continued to crack a smile the whole way home whenever our eyes met.

Exhausted and sunburned, we loaded the canoe to head home.

Home. The word resounded through my mind. I had been in Kapuna about a month now and it was comforting to know I saw it as home.

Just as the engine gained speed across the broad river, I looked up to see a huge rainbow displayed across a cloud. Smiling, I nudged Melanie and pointed. Her face lit up as she instantaneously let out a shriek of delight, clapping her hands. It was God's specific answer to her earlier prayer on the beach. His promises were real.

By this time, everyone on the boat was marveling at the rainbow. The sun went down, as the fading light danced across the rippling rivers. A few hours later we arrived at Kapuna in the dark, exhausted but completely content. True to their welcoming nature, Hanna and Debbie had a hot dinner waiting for all of us. We were home.

CHRISTMAS AT KAPUNA

The culture of Kapuna is a unique one, cultivated out of a mixture of Gulf Province tribal traditions and Judeo-Christian values, meshed with a muddied composition of expats from all over the world—a blending of East and West like no other. One thing is sure, holidays and celebrations are meant for fun and *wantok*.

Coming from a very non-traditional family, I spent a lot of memorable days in the Christmas season at Kapuna. A few days after Christmas, we went around our dinner table sharing stories of our favorite Christmas memories. I had to be honest; Christmas in Kapuna was by far my favorite. I was not likely to forget it any time soon.

Christmas Eve was a flurry of activity. The previous week, staff, students, and patients at the hospital had used paper and food wrappers to create elaborate decorations throughout the wards. Carefully cut and hung, these homemade creations with limited supplies had me marveling at the painstaking, thoughtful work. I had never been a fan of excessive, store bought décor or glittery things. Bush Christmas was much more to my taste. Despite the hot, humid weather, it was hard not to pick up on the spirit of the holiday spreading around.

In her time between ward rounds and patient care, Dr. Beth worked at creating a magnificent gingerbread house. It seemed almost sacrilegious to her nature to not have gingerbread for Christmas festivities. She had the foresight and planned ahead while in Port Moresby, bringing the needed supplies with her.

Only having a few evening hours for the generators to run electricity to our house, she worked through several evenings to bake the walls and roof pieces. The ants and the rats were a constant threat to any of our food items, so she stacked dishes in a pan filled with water, balancing the gingerbread atop it all in a sealed container to preserve it from the critters.

Then, she expertly whipped up multiple icing colors. It came to my attention at the time, that cake baking was an outlet and favorite past time for her. I stood by, in awe of her art. The coconut flakes dyed green made grass, while plain coconut scrapings made snow.

Our baking time was cut short by a Christmas program put on in front of the hospital. The patients and locals lined the veranda. Many songs were sung with the help of torches and headlamps; three children on recorder flutes played as well. Hanna jumped in, adding to the volume of recorder music.

Different groups of children and adults performed skits. Sound systems and lights in the bush are far removed from the huge, thematic productions put on in the first world. If attention to detail and perfection are your preference, you would not appreciate the heart and beauty behind a developing world program. Be prepared for late starts, delays, and equipment fails. The screech of the battery powered speaker and microphone constantly assaulted our ears, as feedback and static came through the microphone—when it actually worked, that is.

Dr. Beth and I rounded up people to join our skit, "Fuddy-Duddy Christmas Cake." The simple yet hilarious, ad-libbed production brought roars of laughter from the crowds. It was mostly physical comedy at its best. One of the community healthcare students later told us she had laughed so hard she almost threw up. With grass stained knees from diving over each other and pain in our ribs from intense laughing, we accepted that compliment with pleasure.

Gerald broke out his hidden musical talents as he played guitar for a group of male students who sang their own rendition of a Christmas hymn.

Another thing one must learn with these types of productions is there is no set ending time. The program can go on for hours and hours. Sometimes half the time is spent waiting for the groups to get ready. Many do not arrive prepared and in costume. Patience was a constant learning objective for my fast-paced, organized Western nature. At the same time, it was one of my favorite things about living in Papua New Guinea. No one was bound by rigorous schedules and a need to be other places at any immediate time. One learns to enjoy things as they come.

Beth and I, however, had an urgency to get back to our house to finish a late night of baking.

The night before Christmas in our bush house, all creatures were stirring, most likely even a mouse. Beth's tasty house was finished but she had a load of gingerbread cookies still to bake. I had my grandmother's brownies to create, as well as a load of my perfected jungle rolls. A confession: they were just basic bread rolls I had mastered in my constant bread making.

Because we only had a toaster oven to bake in, Beth and I kept the extra trays filled with our next food item ready to pop in and out of the oven. The smells emitted from our home likely rivaled any bakery across the world.

In the meantime, the roosters of Kapuna were facing the worst night of their lives. The male students, along with Julian and Gerald, pursued and killed many of the unfortunate poultry. The late night rooster hunt was a traditional event providing protein as a Christmas gift for the hospital patients and families in the area.

After their hunt and slaughter, Julian and Gerald shouted from below our deck to come up for a visit. Stumbling up our stairs, they appeared exhausted but exhilarated, not ready for bed yet. Smelling the baking brownies, they positioned themselves on our deck, waiting for the chance to "clean" the mixing bowl. In the meantime, they shared about the feats of their hunt, testosterone flowing through their veins.

I had to laugh as I listened. Guys will be guys, German, Cantonese, or Papua New Guinean. Their enthusiasm over killing chickens made me glad they enjoyed one of the accomplishments of a well-conditioned bushman.

After taste-testing the freshly baked brownies, they joined Beth and grabbed spoons. In a matter of minutes, every molecule of chocolate batter from the bowl was gone. I pointed out the chocolate around their lips and smeared on their faces.

My prideful nature, when it comes to baking, cannot think of anything better than people thoroughly enjoying my food, especially in a place where it really is a treat.

After the guys returned home for bed, Beth and I remained in our kitchen, trying to keep pace before the second generator turned off at 2 a.m. We wrapped Christmas gifts for secret angels and hospital patients between our toaster oven loads. Once again, I was grateful for Beth's foresight in bringing wrapping paper and cello tape to the jungle. She had even made Christmas cards, which she generously let me use.

I still struggled to believe it was truly Christmas. Wearing nothing but a light dress, I was sweating in the middle of the night, listening to the calls of tropical birds. It was only my second Christmas in the Southern Hemisphere, and my first one not in a Western culture bombarded with commercialism.

Finally, pouring my exhausted body into my bed just as the generator turned off, I drifted into deep sleep.

The chickens were quieter Christmas morning, probably still traumatized by the previous night's hunt. Still, the chance to sleep in was nonexistent. We were gathering at the church around 9 a.m., which in island time translates to an hour or so before we actually finished our morning routines and made our way there.

As we rose and made a quick breakfast and coffee, Beth and I had the brilliant idea of showering the guys with "snow." Of course, the snow really just consisted of a handful of white flour. All of us ex-patriots had been talking of snow a few days before. Most of us hailed from cold climates; however, the New Zealanders and Australian were used to warm weather this season. We dreamed and joked of what Kapuna would look like blanketed in snow. When it rained, we decided it was just melted snow coming down.

Gerald and Julian were accompanied by a group of the young PNG men who had come home from high school on break as they walked to the church on Christmas morning. Due to the lack of higher level schools in the area, once a teen reaches a certain age, around grade eight, they either finish with school or go live in places like Port Moresby with extended family. All of the young men and women were now back with their families for the break.

Gerald and Julian were at the head of the group, so I gingerly tip-toed around the young men making signals for them to be quiet. They caught on to my intentions and smiled. Once at the front of the pack, I shouted, "Happy Christmas!" jubilantly throwing the flour in the air.

Right at that moment, a gust of wind picked up and the majority of the flour flew directly back onto me. The guys had just a small dusting on their heads and shoulders.

I laughed heartily, especially at my own folly, but received a glare in return. Turns out, some humor is not international. These were lessons I was constantly learning.

Upon arrival to the church, I felt like less of a jerk for throwing flour when Debbie arrived. She had a hidden stash of baby powder with which she would attack those she loved most, coating them in the white substance. Throughout the entire Christmas service, someone was bound to fall victim to her pranks.

Decorated from top to bottom with festive balloons and tropical foliage, the church building was a hub of joy. Patients, staff, and students packed the building. Breaking out hymn books, the male students led us in a cappella singing of traditional Christmas songs. The words had been changed and simplified to make more sense in a remote, jungle context with English as a second language. However, not realizing this at first, I loudly belted out the wrong words. Having sung in choir for most of my childhood, as a flame to a struck match, the lyrics flooded my memory.

Finally, we sang some traditional Scot and Irish ballads, sending Debbie and I into a stomping, clapping, and twirling frenzy. Others soon picked up on our sporadic dance and joined in. The youth put on the program with a short message.

Then, our secret angel gifts were handed out. The people of the Gulf region gave with one of the most generous spirits.

The best was still yet to come. Shortly after returning home, Lucy, one of the hospital staff and our neighbor, shyly handed Dr. Beth and me gifts wrapped in notebook paper. Her letter brought me to tears and then I opened my gift, a meri blouse. This dress (or top) is the common style worn currently by PNG women and had red and yellow tropical flowers covering the black fabric Completely functional and appropriate for the conservative village life; it covers shoulders with short puffed sleeves and hangs loosely down to the knees.

I quickly changed out of my clothes and put it on. I finally felt converted to a *bush-meri* (bush woman).

We assembled for the feast at the Treehouse where Robbie and Debbie, along with Melanie and Hanna, lived. The Calvert family shortly joined the rest of us, as the spread on the table kept growing. It was all traditional meals amended to meet the provisions of the swamp lands.

Debbie had made stuffing inside a pumpkin, warning us that she was missing some of the sewing pins that had held the gourd together during the baking process.

Hanna brilliantly created a nativity scene out of clothes pegs. Their little wooden smiling faces looked back at us from their hand-crafted cloth outfits. Sheep were fashioned from tufts of polyester stuffing, and baby Jesus laid to rest at the center, placed in a miniature baby bilum.

Treats like Coke and chocolate finally made their appearance, along with traditional Christmas crackers that popped and revealed cheap plastic toys and paper crowns. Everything was a delight in the midst of our usually simplistic lifestyle.

Around the crowded table, eight nationalities were represented. In Maori, Spanish, German, French, Chinese, and Pidgin, we recited Luke 2:11.

The Christmas past of commercialism and gaudy decorations was completely replaced in my mind by this entirely delightful Christmas present. It was a time to celebrate with people I loved, who had become my family and closest friends. We filled ourselves on the wonderful food and relished happy conversation and joy, united in our love for Papua New Guinea and our faith.

That evening, regretting our overly-full stomachs and food comas, we lounged around on chairs and mattresses.

A death adder almost put a damper on our festivities. The previous few days, dead chickens had been found in the garden. The only explanation: a snake. The downstairs neighbor, Cyril, appeared in the doorway while we basked in our lethargy. One look at the solemnity across his usually smiling countenance told us he had something vital to share. He had beheaded the deadly snake under the treehouse. The warning was clear; take a torch and watch where you walk through the grasses. Another reminder that nature should be respected in PNG. Christmas day was just another day to a death adder.

BAT THE RAT

While the festivities of Christmas were about uniting in the joy and love of our Savior, New Year's Eve was the holiday that resurrected the child in each of us. Kapuna was a place that consistently seemed brimming with delight and a reason to celebrate.

At dinner, Dr. Beth was asked to pop an obscene amount of popcorn. It was not an easy task done over a wood burning stove. We filled a plastic baby bath with the fluffy kernels. It was the end prize for a scavenger hunt put together by the students.

Per usual, when we entered the church that evening, only a handful of people had gathered at the appointed time. Seeing rolled-up newspaper sticks and a ball of newspaper, Auntie Barb challenged Gerald and Julian to a man versus woman game of "Bat the Rat," essentially hockey with newspaper.

Next thing I knew, in a blurry haze of sprinting back and forth across the church floor, diving, hitting, and near-tackles, the four of us competed to get goals. My severely competitive nature was starting to show itself as I shoved past Gerald, who had boxed me out. Ignoring my urges to hit him with my rolled up newspaper, I skidded across the floor, finally hitting the paper "rat" into the goal to score our winning point.

Bruised and sweaty, we finished our game as the majority of the attendees had now shown up.

Gasping for breath, we looked at each other and laughed over the intensity of the game.

A schedule of games followed the scavenger hunt with another version of "bat the rat" which included about thirty of us rotating in and out. Hospital patients joined staff and students, all enjoying the evening immensely. My night was made complete, however, by the game of flashlight hide-and-seek.

Armed with torches and tennis balls, the finders counted as a number of us scattered into the dark area seeking a place of refuge. I crouched in thigh high, damp grass with Sekpain as we waited for the bouncing torchbearers to come near us. My only prayer, at that time, was that no snakes would be joining us for the game. As the lights made their way closer, we sprinted from shadow to shadow in the pineapple patch, eluding their searching eyes. I finally made a break and darted to the base, hurling myself over the railing and to safety just as a seeker rounded the corner.

Since I was a small child, hide-and-seek has been my favorite. I played as if my life truly depended on not being found. I remember frightening babysitters after long searches when they were fruitless in finding me. I would then emerge as I heard panic crack in their voices as they called for me.

Needless to say, I was having the time of my life with everyone else. I saw the same youthful glow in the eyes of Dr. Valerie and Auntie Barb as they joined us for the games. The night transcended cultural barriers and age. It was another lesson reminding me of the equal value of all lives regardless of nationality, culture, belief, or financial status.

Exhausted and sweat stained, we headed home to shower and prepare for midnight.

Freshly clean, I reemerged with my headlamp, following the path to the front of the hospital. Most of the patients had returned to their villages for the holidays or had gone to bed after the games, so the gathering was sparse. A staff member played songs on his guitar under the stars, and we joined in.

Then, a giant pile of wood and palm fronds was lit. An almost instantaneous heat met us as the dry kindling created an inferno. It sent dancing sparks into the night sky. We cheered. The New Year was here. Finally, paper lanterns were lit, rising over the swamp and drifting down river toward Ara'ava.

Exhausted, we headed to bed passing shouts of the younger people still running around and celebrating. This was home. One year earlier, I never would have imagined I would ring in the New Year in one of the most remote places on earth. Gratitude filled my heart. There was no place I would rather be. Kapuna was my greatest blessing for the holidays.

Auntie Barb's sweet spirit and love of creating festivities was a gift, because the daily life and realities of the Gulf Province were sometimes hard to face, especially the illness and death that came in the form of tuberculosis.

TUBERCULOSIS

Emaciated bodies, wracked with coughing, fever, and night sweats are some obvious physical indicators of tuberculosis (TB). While TB is preventable and curable, it still affects millions of people each year. According to the World Health Organization, at least 1.3 million people died from TB in 2012.

It is a disease that does not have preferences but impacts the young, old, female, and male alike.

In remote areas like the Gulf Province of Papua New Guinea, TB can be difficult to track, diagnose, and treat. Availability and capacity of facilities add to the problem. The Gulf Province only has three hospitals. Understanding of this invisible killer is also difficult to articulate throughout the remote regions. Many patients, despite the doctors' warnings, abscond before their treatment ends creating an even worse problem: drug resistant TB.

Dr. Patrick shared one memorable story of a father's dedication to save his son. As an only child, the beautiful three year old was clearly loved by his doting father. After a few days of illness, his boy became increasingly drowsy and had a high fever. Traveling four days nonstop during the rainy season, the father paddled down with the tide. The boy's condition worsened with each hour. With only twelve hours to get to Kikori, the little boy started to convulse. He was unconscious by the time they made it.

Dr. Patrick diagnosed the little guy with meningitis and TB. They put a tube in his stomach and began to treat him. It did not look promising; the toddler was in a coma. Never leaving his side, the father was distressed.

Thanks to the effort of the staff and the great love of the father, the little boy gained consciousness two days later. Within three weeks, he was back on his feet. Patrick said it was clear the little boy was adored and his father took good care of him. He was confident this parent would finish his child's treatment and therefore fully recover.

Unfortunately, for every victory, there are many children who never make it to the hospital. Patrick says there are patients who travel three days by foot from the highlands. Sheer determination and resilience keeps them going.

Since awareness and education about illness is vital to stopping the spread of disease, the Kikori staff started movie nights. Drawn in with the promise of a film, the patients and locals are forced to learn more about medical conditions in order to watch an entertaining flick. It seems so simple, but teaching to prevent the spread of TB is the difference of life or death for thousands in the Gulf Province.

A BOY CALLED ROMAN

As I high-fived the tiny, claw-like hand, I took in the emaciated five year old's wide grin. He was an enthusiastic, talkative child from the Gulf Province. Roman's ribs protruded and his arms and legs could not support his meager weight. He was suffering from severe, drug-resistant tuberculosis. Yet, he was a miracle sitting in front of me.

When he arrived at the bush hospital five months earlier, the medical staff had battled for his life, knowing it was against all odds. Roman possesses an undefinable quality, making him special, making him a survivor. Everyone loved him dearly. Who could resist his lively greetings, broad smile, and waving arms?

Looking at Roman's thin frame, I am transported back to over a year ago on my first trip to PNG and another little boy, Wesley, the three year old I met in Bamio.

His mother had come to the clinic to see if we could help her son. One look at the little guy and I knew he was on the brink of death. His little knees were bigger than his thighs. The left side of his body was slack, unused. His large eyes followed my face. Staring seemed to be all he had strength to do.

Having little knowledge of TB, I just thought the child was starving to death. Now I know he was in the last phases of the horrible disease. The doctors examined him but knew little could be done. The nearest hospital was days away via canoe.

The memory of him, however, is etched deeply upon my life. His existence was short. He lived in a remote, unknown corner of the world, but Wesley changed everything for me.

That little boy was key to why I returned to PNG.

Now, I met Roman.

Roman is special to all of us in Kapuna. Roman is living the story I wish Wesley could have lived. Roman is living.

I look at his big smile, feel the touch of his hand, and I know we are headed in the right direction. I am grateful for his spirit. I am grateful for Kapuna Hospital working hard to treat patients in the remote bush. He reminds me this is how I want to spend my life, making the marginalized unforgettable, making sure they are loved.

After I left Kapuna, Dr. Beth informed me Roman had finished his treatment and returned home. She was happy for his recovery. I knew Roman was also one of her favorites. Having seen him every day for so long, I was pretty sure Beth would have kept him forever if she could.

THE REALITY OF SORCERY

Darkness encroaches. Aroused by the noise outside, sleeping villagers rub their bleary eyes and poke their heads out of their homes. Pulses quickening, they watch as a mob passes close by. Every single time this happens, it is terrifying. Yet it is part of the fabric of the culture. Witch hunts have been going on for generations, possibly a few thousand years.

Both Papua New Guinean and international media have exploded with accounts of violence associated with sorcery in the highlands. Places like Mt. Hagen and Goroka recently experienced such an influx of vigilante justice. They blamed witchcraft for the violence. It compounded to the point that many people had to stop traveling through, for fear of their lives. Work in surrounding areas came to a grinding halt because people refused to leave their homes, or pass through certain sections of town. Sometimes it carried on for days, sometimes much longer.

In April 2013, Prime Minister Peter O'Neill called for the nation to repeal an act that protected violence against accused witchcraft. Despite this, the nation is taking a pelting from groups like Amnesty International, who claim repealing the act was not enough to protect the rights and lives of those accused of sorcery. Their aim was mostly targeted at helping women, twisting the focus more towards women's rights than just violence related to sorcery. I don't believe, in my brief experience in PNG, that witch hunts are the sexist acts American groups want to label them; they are rooted in thousands of years of belief, effecting both men and women.

When I asked a couple of students at Kapuna what one of their most memorable hospital stories was, they told a harrowing tale of a victim of a sorcery hunt. He arrived at the hospital with his face almost completely removed.

Speculation will never reveal whether the man truly practiced witchcraft or not. The students I interviewed had not investigated his true religious practices. It appeared after the brutal attack from villagers, someone took pity on the man, bringing him via canoe. When the patient was brought to Kapuna Hospital in the dead of the night after a mob attempted to remove all of the skin from his face, he was looked after and treated as anyone else who would come through the doors. The doctor, nurses, and students worked quickly to repair the knife wounds. He was barely conscious, having lost excessive amounts of blood.

"Doctor [Valerie] sutured everything back again. He is okay now, but he was here for a while," Theophilla stated. The community healthcare workers shared the story as if it were just another day at the job. They said the doctor stitched his face back together, after repairing other vital knife wounds. Sekpain nodded in agreement as Theophilla shared. They were both there when the man was brought in. I wondered to what extent of "okay" the students meant. After all, in Papua New Guinean terms it could likely mean, he survived without severe infection. My imagination could do little in understanding the extent of agony and scarring the man had gone through. Without cosmetic surgery and performed with limited resources, surgery was based more on saving a life and staving off infection than looking attractive. Of course, the doctors tried to reduce scaring and restore the body as much as possible.

Both community healthcare workers have been witness to many atrocities done by and done to witch doctors. Sorcery is part of life in the bush. Outsiders, especially from Western nations, tend to attribute it simply to jealousy and socio-economic situations. An article written on June 10, 2013 by the Associated Press tells the story of Helen Rumbali. After a mob stormed her home by night, they burned it to the ground, dragging her and others off to be tortured. Tragically, she was beheaded in the process.

The article states:

A wealth of mineral resources and natural gas has transformed the nation's long-stagnant economy into one of the world's fastest growing over the past decade, increasing on average almost 7 percent annually from 2007 to 2010. Growth peaked at 8.9 percent in 2011 before slowing to 8 percent last year.

The Asian Development Bank reported last year that Papua New Guinea has one of the highest levels of inequality, if not the highest, in the Asia-Pacific region.

These socio-economic problems have inevitably played into a cultural landscape that includes a belief in witches and black magic, said Kate Schuetze, a regional researcher for Amnesty International.

"There is always a reason for the accusation, whether it's jealousy, wanting to access someone else's land, a personal grudge against that person or a previous land dispute," Schuetze said.

Dr. Patrick shared an instance of this. I asked him to tell me a story about his most memorable patients.

In a small village situated in the Southern Highlands near the Gulf Province boarder, Wemono and her youngest son, Charlie, crouched in the darkness and rain unsure if they would live to see the morning. Trembling uncontrollably, the fear of that night raced through their minds. It had happened so quickly. Conflict had arisen after a few cows in the village died of inexplicable causes. Villagers blamed it on sorcery and needed someone to pin it on. It did not take long for accusations of black magic against the cows to fall on Wemono. There had been suspicions of jealousy.

A mob carrying axes, machetes, and knives charged Wemono's home as dusk set in. Hearing noise, sixteen-year-old Charlie rushed outside and confronted the horde. Despite his incredible bravery, his small stature was no match for the brute force against him. Men swung at him with their weapons. An ax almost completely severed his shoulder, gashing into the bone. The chopping and stabbing soon took him down.

Motherly instinct kicking in, Wemono abandoned all sense of self-preservation and ran out to defend her son. She too fell victim to multiple stab wounds. Still alive, but severely wounded, they ran to safety in the confines of the dense jungle nearby. Unsure if their home was still standing or had been looted, they fled into the night. They waited near the highway connecting the highlands to Kikori. Both bled profusely.

Finally, long after dawn had broken and the sun was almost at its peak, a vehicle emerged in the distance. Both were on the verge of going into shock.

Unaware, the road construction crew lumbered down the highway when they saw the two on the side of the road. Stopping, the men put Wemono and Charlie in the back of their truck and headed toward Kikori Hospital. Along the way they made one more stop to pick up a young girl who had been attacked in a separate incident and left to bleed to death.

Dr. Patrick was alerted that evening, as the patients arrived to the hospital. All of the nurses and medical staff were there to stabilize all three victims at once. The young woman was in shock. The hospital team got drips into each patient. Working through the night, they stitched up the wounds.

Dr. Patrick grew close to the patients in their two month stay. He said despite their persecution, they had fantastic attitudes. Horrible infection set in, so they were bed ridden for a while. He indicated the pain they endured was unimaginable. As they healed, they would sit up chatting with the staff or take walks around the hospital grounds. Once more mobile, the duo would bring him food throughout the day. Charlie's arm eventually regained some mobility.

Patrick laughed as he recounted Wemono joking about her youngest son. She had many older sons and every single one of them was a kick boxer and very strong, except for small

Charlie. He was the youngest and weakest, yet his bravery spoke volumes about his character. With a humorous twinkle in her eye, she lamented that of all the sons to be home at the time of the attack, it had to be Charlie. The doctor was pretty convinced by the end of their stay that the attacks were out of spite. He had trouble believing the sweet, motherly Wemono was a witch.

There is merit to what many outside experts have to say. After all, the Western world can draw from its own history and experience. The famous Salem Witch Trials in the late 1600s are a thread in the early history of the North American Colonies. Research by historians has shown a link to jealousy of property and landownership disputes.

Mass hysteria and mob mentality fanned the flames of witch hunts and accusations. Europe can trace similar historical events, but all of them go deeper into not only property disputes but different religious uprisings at the time.

With the telling and retelling of history, however, Europeans and North Americans may miss that there were threads of truth about sorcery woven into the complications of the times. Much like Papua New Guinea, the issues are more profound than an either-or option. History in the American Colonies also reveals a rooted belief in the supernatural. Facts remain that there was practice of witchcraft.

If you talk to the locals, regardless of the people group or region, you will hear very different tales than the Western media would attribute. I have yet to meet one who has not been witness to acts of sorcery. The Melanesian people have roots and practices in animism. I personally have met a few witchdoctors in villages I visited in the Western Province.

"Sorcery affects treatment here a lot," Sekpain and Theophilla stated. They went on to explain it not only affects the hospital receiving victims from the violence against alleged witches, it also affects the type of treatment people in the area choose to pursue.

Held captive by animism, superstition, and a lack of medical knowledge, many villagers will seek treatment by local witch doctors rather than go to a healthcare worker or the hospital. Often times their treatment is a mixture of both, usually when one fails to produce desired results. Because science and knowledge of disease is not widely taught or known, illness and disease can be attributed to the spiritual realm. Therefore, patients seek spiritual cures for their disease.

Of course, I am not quick to merely dismiss or minimize their beliefs. Not all people will agree, but I believe as a Christian that there is an element to our world and life that is spiritual and does need consideration and understanding.

I witnessed and photographed a baptismal ceremony that demonstrated the clear existence of witchcraft in the local spiritual culture.

A local woman in her forties wearing a solemn look stood waist deep in the murky water. A woman on her right and one on her left asked about her commitment to follow Christ. Inaudible talking ensued. She stared into the water, taking in the words.

Gathered at the water's edge, the crowd waited breathlessly in the significance of this moment. I was crouched in tall grasses on the banks, focusing my camera on her face. The grass tickled my legs but I hardly noticed over the anticipation of her words. Raising her voice for all to hear, the woman declared that she decided to make Jesus Christ the Lord of her life. She set aside her former practices of witchcraft, recognizing them as an opposition to God.

Cheers rose from all around as the women on either side of the former sorceress dunked her in the water, baptizing her in the name of the Father, the Son, and the Holy Spirit. A guitar strummed as the congregation began singing. Having risen from the water, the woman smiled for the first time, wiping the beads of water off her face.

In another experience, in another part of PNG, my friend, Effy, told of her experience. She traveled the Sandaun Province of PNG where she experienced the sorcery practices first-hand.

We were staying in a village called Maiynroiyn in the Sissano language area and running our usual kids' program in the afternoon. I was walking to the field where everyone was playing. This old woman stopped me. When she saw me she got the biggest smile on her face. It seemed like she recognized me, like I was a long-lost daughter or relative. She hugged me and was laughing, crying, and nuzzling her face into my neck and shoulder. I was a little overwhelmed by the greeting, but I just figured it had been a really long time since any missionary or white person had been to this village so she must have just been excited or thankful to see me.

For the next day, that little lady became my shadow; she would take me by the arm and walk me around the village, introducing me to everyone and chatting away to me in a mix of Tok Pisin and Sissano. She offered me water, food, and gave me one of the biggest pineapples I have ever seen! The next day was the same until half way through the day. The Wycliffe leader that had been trekking with us and one of our local translators asked to talk to me and pulled me aside. They informed me that the woman who had been hanging around me was actually a witch and that she believed that I was the spirit of her dead daughter whom she had called back to be with her. Needless to say I was a little shocked and was not quite sure what to do next, but God is faithful. We were able to use this not-so-great situation to bring truth to an entire village! Many different people in this village had started to believe this about me so our translator gathered all the people together in the meeting place and was able to talk to them on what the Bible says about death, and life, and spirits. We were able to pray for the village and I was actually able to pray for the witch myself! What an honor to be a part of bringing the truth of who God is to our brothers and sisters in PNG.

Whether jealousy is to blame, or not, is less of an issue. Reality in Papua New Guinea is that witchcraft affects the lives of most villagers in some capacity or another, which plays into their views of Western medicine. With animistic roots, the culture has to come to terms with their expanding knowledge of the sciences and medicine, along with the spread of the Christian faith. It also, unfortunately, leaves people with an excuse to do harm to their neighbor or property.

VILLAGE LIFE IN WOWOBO

While the doctor and hospital staff worked in the busy clinics, I took my camera and wandered down the sloping grasses that overlooked the Purari River. Wowobo is situated at a distinct bend in the river. The vibrant blue sky and cumulous clouds reflected almost perfectly off the calm waters next to the muddy banks below. The Gulf Province boasted some of the most incredible skyline I had ever viewed.

Wowobo was my favorite village so far. Meandering hills were dotted with the huts and an array of tropical vegetation. During rainy season, the packed dirt and sloping hillsides must be a nightmare to navigate, but here in the dry season it was a romantic little spot in the Gulf Province, romantic-looking enough to almost induce me to throw off all of my American ideals and settle down in a thatched hut with a little garden, never to return to my Western life.

I'm still tempted.

As I neared the children playing on the grassy hillside, they hit the ball to me. The game was simple enough. There was an old tennis ball. You could kick it, hit it, or throw it. The goal was just to keep it off the ground. The children were quite skilled at it. I joined them in a round of giggles as we chased the ball all over the hillside, hitting it to one another. More and more kids joined in. So much for not getting too sweaty!

Thirst and mild exhaustion set in, so I walked further down the hill to where the adults sat. Right below them was a steep grade that ended at the waterfront. My eyes fell on a young girl, probably in her pre-teen years. She was holding a beautiful, perfectly chubby baby with a dirty skirt on. The baby's glossy dark eyes met mine and my heart melted. I am starting to understand what love at first sight means.

I had barely reached my hands out to hold the baby, when the baby reached for me. I snatched her up in my arms and proceeded to cuddle her. In an instant we were connected. Curious, the chubby, slobbery hands went for the camera around my neck. She was intrigued by all of the buttons. I talked to her softly, showing her in the simplest terms how to use my camera.

I then scooped her up, lifted her in the air and jiggled her lightly. She squealed with delight. Her big smile revealed her little teeth popping through. We continued this for several minutes.

I now understood how stay-at-home mothers could spend their entire day, completely revolved around a little person. This baby was amazing! Everything she did made me smile.

The local adults were more entertained by my love for this baby than I think they were by the elated grins and noises she produced. As I played with the baby, I tried to engage the adults around me. They barely spoke English and I had no knowledge of their local language, but we bonded. One woman was able to tell me enough.

The young girl holding the baby was the older sister. Their mother, who was probably not much older than me, had just died. They were not sure what her illness was, just that it was sudden. Four children were left motherless. The baby was still nursing, so a nearby woman indicated she was providing milk.

I wondered how this woman could nurse her two small children in her lap, plus provide for the sweet little one in my lap. I was grateful, however, that the village cared enough for these children to sacrifice for them.

It broke my heart to think of the glowing, big eyes that met mine and know she would never know her mom. I wondered if a kind woman, who loved to cuddle this little one, would one day take the mother's place or if this baby would grow up without those important ministrations.

I was relieved when I met the grandmother, who smiled gently at her *booboo* (grandchild). After a long period of more play and cuddles, I reluctantly handed the baby over. She immediately whimpered and tears filled her eyes. I felt her pain; I did not want to part either.

The grandmother placed her back in my arms and she calmed down. I cuddled some more, talking to her gently. As it was time to move on, I placed the baby this time in her sister's arms. Our scene repeated as tears filled her eyes.

I had to walk away.

She broke into a wail.

My heart broke as I left the motherless baby. I knew she was loved. It made it a little better.

Later I pondered what it must be like as a dying mother. I cannot imagine having to say a final goodbye to these darling children. Did she wonder how they would do without her? I hoped she knew how cared for they were.

It was a reminder that in the midst of this tropical paradise, healthcare was still in great need. Mothers and children are dying at alarming rates of curable and treatable diseases.

Just in this village alone we saw many cases of tuberculosis, ulcers, malnutrition, and even leprosy. My prayer is that this will change. That people will care enough about this corner of the world to spend their lives serving and making medical improvements. Maybe one day, the cuddly, sweet babies will not have to lose their parents.

This is my prayer.

THE HELICOPTER RIDE

After unemployment had left Pase John unable to properly provide for his family, he left Lae in Morobe Province. As he searched, Pase was led to the Gulf Province where he found a temporary job with an oil and mineral company, building bridges. The labor was hard, but he was happy to work for his wife and young children.

A gentle smile crossed his serious face when he talked about his small boy and baby girl. Sadness shone in his eyes, as well. He had not been in contact with them for months. It was hard to stay in touch when he was at his work camp in a remote area.

Laboring on the bridges for a few months, the days wore into weeks, and life was in a bit of a rhythm with nothing much changing. Then, what started as an ordinary week of hard labor changed dramatically as he began to feel weak—weaker than his usual fatigue.

Both of his upper arms were losing strength at an alarming rate. That night, he tried to rest well. When he awoke on the Wednesday morning and got out of bed, his arms remained limp and now his legs were being drained of all strength.

Pase, like many Papua New Guinean men, was not tall but he had an imposing strength. His lean muscle indicated a life of demanding toil.

Doubts flickered through his mind as the extreme exhaustion came on. He knew something was wrong; this was beyond pure weariness. He alerted the base camp medic, who brushed off Pase's concern. After a brief medical examination, Pase was sent back to his bed.

Pase awoke in the night with a terrifying revelation. Try as he might, he could not move a muscle. Although he could talk, he was completely paralyzed. Panic set in as he called for help.

By the time the medical staff was alerted, they were sure Pase was dead. His heart rate was barely registering. Not a muscle moved.

That morning, they rushed him to their base camp in Tuel where they attempted to stabilize the dying man. Isaac Anley, the base paramedic, took over. He knew there was not much they could do and they needed to get Pase to a hospital as soon as possible if saving him were even feasible.

With the helicopter blades rotating swiftly overhead, Pase was strapped in with Isaac by his side. They took off and made the couple-hour flight via chopper to the bush hospital in Kapuna.

Mid-Thursday morning, the Kapuna staff had done their rounds in the wards. Many of them were sitting in the living room of Dr. Lin, Grandma, enjoying devotions. The singing had ended and it was more of a time of conversation when the tell-tale resonance of a distant helicopter broke the normal jungle noises. It was the second helicopter to arrive that week.

The doctors had been busy the past few days with an influx of severe tuberculosis patients; although this was a fairly normal state for Kapuna hospital to be in. As the helicopter broke through the dense grey clouds in the morning sky, they knew there was likely another emergency to handle.

Since most patients—even extremely sick ones—usually arrived via canoe or dinghy, flights in are reserved for many of the worst cases.

The staff dispersed from their devotions and headed to the pad that sat amidst the swampy grasses in front of the hospital. Patients, families, and students all came running, clamoring close enough to see the metal beast with its swiftly rotating arms. Isaac jumped out. Aided by staff, he carried Pase into the hospital.

The doctors were at a loss as to why a healthy, 26-year-old man would wake up paralyzed with a diminishing heart rate. ECG's showed the heart rate was at risk of completely stopping. After a round of checks and basic diagnostic testing, Dr. Valerie and Dr. Beth diagnosed low potassium and treated to stabilize him. Then they, and even retired Dr. Lin, went off to consult every resource they could find to figure out why it was so low.

THE PRAYER

Haunted by the terrified gaze of the dying man, they prayed as they worked.

Dr. Beth said, "His desperate look met my panicked one as I sent up probably the shortest but most effective prayer I have ever prayed, 'God, HELP'."

As research and reading ensued, the three women came back together to discuss their findings. Dr. Beth found the diagnosis in books, and Grandma reminded Valerie that she had seen it once before as a student. (What a wonderful memory 89-year-old Dr. Lin has!) All of them had come to the same diagnostic conclusion: Shakhonovich's syndrome . . . Hypokalaemic periodic paralysis. It was the only diagnosis that made sense with the failing heart rate.

The disease is genetic and very rare, usually showing itself in adolescence. Potassium, which helps muscles and maintains the heartbeat, does not transfer properly between membranes. This causes extreme muscle weakness when potassium levels drop or in extreme cases complete paralysis. If not treated timely the heart can stop.

The other risk of the disease is that recovery is quick and almost instantaneous. The sudden high potassium in the blood adversely affects the heart rhythm and can cause fatal arrhythmias. The patient has to be closely monitored to ensure this does not happen.

Days later, they asked Pase what was going on in his head as all of this was happening. He said initially just terror. He did not think he would ever see his family again. Due to the remoteness and suddenness of his illness, his family was completely unaware of his condition throughout the ordeal.

He said once he was in the care of the doctors, and could sense their concern, and had all of the tests running, his fear eased a bit. He knew they were doing everything possible for him.

Slowly they watched his heart rate improve with the potassium treatment.

Thursday felt like an eternity in the eyes of Pase and the staff at Kapuna.

By Friday morning, Pase was more assured by the doctors. Isaac never left his side, as he interpreted the English into Tok Pisin for the young man.

Monitoring him closely in case his potassium levels spiked, the waiting game for his sudden recovery began.

THE LAME CAN WALK

Friday evening Dr. Beth did her usual rounds. While checking on Pase, he complained to her of pain in his chest. She prayed it would not be something worse and asked him where his pain was located. Without thinking, he lifted his hand and pointed to the source of the pain.

Dr. Beth, Pase, and Isaac all realized in that moment Pase was recovering.

Pase could move his hand and arms. His feeling and strength were returning. Overjoyed, they waited breathlessly to see how much he could do physically. In less than an hour, the patient sat up and swung his legs over the edge of his bed. With shaky steps, he began to walk across the room.

After monitoring his heart to make sure it was stabilized, Dr. Beth left her healed paralysis patient in joy and informed Dr. Valerie and those around the hospital of his recovery. Face alight, she came to us friends, to inform us of the miraculous healing.

Our cheers could probably be heard a long way off.

We all knew it was moments like this that kept the medical staff going. It made the hard work and sleepless nights worth it.

It's not every day a person can say they saw a paralyzed man get up and walk. The staff at Kapuna can. It happened thanks to the hard work of a dedicated medical staff, the wisdom of God, and the determination of a man to live!

THE DAY THE CANOE SANK

Another morning, awakened early by the chickens, I decided to go into the office early to get extra work done. As I walked along the worn path, I saw Gerald in a rush leaving Colin and Barb's house where he was staying while they were away. He had a panicked look on his face as he passed me.

"The canoe sank!" He said, hustling to the office.

Trying to remain calm for a few split seconds I envisioned the Calverts, Ben, Dr. Patrick, and crew stranded and wet on some muddy embankment as their boat slowly sank to the bottom of a river, bubbles gurgling to the surface after it went down. I snapped back to reality. I quickly followed behind him into the building. Thankfully Gerald saw the panic on my face, stopped, and clarified that it had been docked when it sank.

"How did you even find out? Wait, what exactly happened?" I fumbled over my words trying to comprehend the situation.

One of the hospital staff awoke Gerald early that morning telling him the canoe had sunk. Having the same vision I did, he was not fully awake and imagined our *wantok* drowned. It was pure PNG communication style to tell the absolute most shocking information first and then fill in the details. After

Gerald got his heart started again, the staff member explained the canoe had not been tied up to the dock properly overnight when it sank.

The group had stopped at a few villages on their way to Kikori Hospital. They spent the previous day doing clinics. Planning to spend the night in the village, they had tied up the boat on a low tide and went to bed. Unfortunately, as the tide was rising, the canoe swung under a dock. The waters continued to come up, but the boat was trapped. Eventually it filled with water and sank. When the team rose in the morning to continue their journey, they found the discouraging news. Dragging it off of the river floor, they emptied it. The outboard motor was water logged. They had to dry it out before testing to see if it worked. The Gulf Province has very patchy cell phone service, so it was a miracle their phone was able to call Kapuna's security office that morning.

Caught up with the situation, Gerald ran to his computer to Skype with Uncle John, the Aussie mechanic who served in Kapuna a few months a year. Uncle John was sending him detailed instructions on fixing the outboard.

"What can I do to help?" I asked, knowing the guys quickly had to get a dinghy loaded and ready for a rescue mission.

While Gerald rounded up staff and prepared to leave, I ran around printing instructions and gathering food and water for their journey. The guys had to be prepared for the possibility that the water-logged outboard would not start. They might be gone for a few days running people back to Kikori and bringing Kapuna's staff back. In the midst of the chaotic rush, I had to stop and laugh. Never could I have imagined this would be my life. The Land of the Unexpected again lived up to its name.

Gerald and I prayed for the motor to be fixed. The rescue dinghy then left. I had to trust it would all be alright. It was now about lunch time, so I resumed my work. So much for getting extra work done. With little to no ability to communicate with the team, Grandma, Dr. Beth, and I would just have to wait until everyone returned to get the full story.

Later in the day, we received a phone call from Kikori Hospital informing us they were limping home with a slow motor but would make it that evening. Family dinner was a little dull as Grandma and I ate our usual cooked bananas, boiled greens, and pumpkin, watching the sun set, hoping the boats would find their way home safely after dark.

In the end, everything worked out alright. It was another lesson on the difficulties this region had to overcome.

THE MIRACLE OF MEDICINE

Kapuna Hospital manages to treat tens of thousands of people over the years. Despite the incredibly hard work and knowledge of the staff, they are limited by their lack of resources. Until recently, there was no good, working ultrasound. The x-ray machine had been in disrepair for years, parts were hard to come by and technicians to fix it did not exist. As far as laboratories go, the humidity melts test papers, rendering them useless.

The lab is literally an old microscope set up in the office with dirty slides. We did learn how to spot tuberculosis on a slide. I am constantly held in awe of how the doctors can do so much with so few resources, so I was not surprised when one day this issue imploded.

It was January. The monthly shipment of medicine had not come in, nor the previous months'. The barge that usually brought it never arrived. The doctors contacted their suppliers. No one seemed to know what happened to the medication.

Surely it was sitting in a warehouse somewhere in Port Moresby, expiring in the intense heat and humidity, or dropped at a wrong location in another hospital, wasting in a storeroom somewhere. Regardless of the medicines' incredulous fate, Kapuna Hospital was in want.

Frustrations mounted. They were literally down to their last few bottles of ibuprofen, a basic painkiller. How does a doctor treat patients without medicine?

Patients who should be on morphine were being meted out the few remaining pills. Only the desperate, worst cases would get these simple medications. Among those who did qualify were a woman with a broken spine and a patient with cancer. These were the worst cases. The staff passed by several sufferers, unable to offer respite. They were down to three bottles for over 100 patients. For those who already spent their lives without little access to medical care, this was too much. No one had any idea when the next shipment was due to arrive, if it would even turn up. The situation was more than grim.

Empty storeroom shelves taunted the staff as they passed the pharmacy.

Within twelve hours of the doctors' complete despair over the medicine, people from around the world began to message the doctors online, letting them know they were praying fervently for our corner of the bush.

With no solution except prayer, the doctors went to bed and awoke for rounds before church on a Sunday morning.

It started like every Sunday. We rose to the boisterous roosters, shuffled around our homes, and ate breakfast admiring our profusion of wild flowers out front. The clanging of the bell called us all to start moving faster and head to church. Guitars and voices were being tuned. The swell of voices sounded as the church-goers trickled in. Another noise also appeared, growing louder. A large engine caught the attention of everyone all over the village.

Ships never come on Sundays!

Several people left their posts and sprinted to the jetty. Kids yelled and waved, unsure of what they celebrated. In front of Kapuna, the ship cut its engine. Unaware of what was going on, the staff passed boxes that were being handed down the line. More and more boxes appeared without any explanation. Carried to the drug store, the staff opened all the boxes! 36 unexplained boxes of medicine just appeared at the hospital.

Dr. Beth described herself as a kid on Christmas day.

One box housed eight enormous bottles of 1,000 pain relief tablets each. Then, they discovered another. And another. Over and over pain medication and many other needed tablets were being pulled out. In their delight and giddiness, the doctors and nurses paused, comprehending this was not the order they had put in months ago.

After further investigation, it was discovered this was a generic shipment. A routine ship carried these supplies to different health centers around Papua New Guinea one to two times a year.

Call it whatever you deem, but the people at Kapuna do not see mere coincidence in a random ship arriving at the most desperate hour after hundreds of friends around the world prayed for us. We know our minds cannot comprehend the depths of it all, but we believe God heard those prayers and answered in abundance.

It was our miracle; our miracle of medicine.

Reflecting on the day, Dr. Beth shared Ephesians 3:20, "Now to Him who is able to do immeasurably more than all we ask or imagine, according to His power that is at work within us…" In my writing of this book, my desire was to not make it a "Christian book," as that tends to bend toward a select audience and alienate everyone who is not, but when I sat down to write, I knew I could not leave the "God parts" out. Because when I wrote this story, I realized this was not Kapuna's story, or the Calverts' story, or my story, or the people of PNG's story, this is God's story. He is woven into the fabric of life in Kapuna.

He is madly in love with the people of Papua New Guinea and He allows people like the Calverts and Pettersons to love Papua New Guinea with Him. And, they do.

CONCLUSION

I have fallen completely in love with the nation of Papua New Guinea and the people who make up the composition of its story. Like anywhere in the world, Papua New Guinea has its incredibly bright spots as well as some frustrating roadblocks to progress.

I hesitate to tell the story of Kapuna for fear people would want to change so much about PNG. At the same time, I recognize the injustice of remaining silent about maternal mortality rates, children dying of preventable disease, and people, in general, lacking basic sanitation knowledge and capabilities.

My heart in telling this story is to completely honor the people of Papua New Guinea in the midst of building capacity to see healthcare improve. While I viewed PNG with some cultural blinders on, I hope to encourage the readers to fall in love with PNG with me. I hope to bring understanding to their way of life, while also informing people of needs. I have no desire to change PNG or turn it into another Western Culture. There is incredible beauty in our cultural differences, but make no mistake there are hurdles that the resilient, wonderful people of this nation face.

There is a need to see medical care throughout remote PNG improved and needs met. Like anything worth having, this is not easy. If fixing problems like this were simple, it would have already been done. The fact of the matter is, developing communities and improving healthcare affect many facets of society, come in so many different perspectives and solutions, and take time. Time is not something many in the Western world care to invest.

This book will not solve the problems, but I hope it encourages people to seek solutions and get involved. I am blessed to know so many people through organizations like Youth with a Mission, Mission Aviation Fellowship, New Tribes, Summer Institute of Linguistics, Gulf Christian Services, and the Papua New Guinea government who are there making a difference, living it out each day.

I want their lives to be living proof it is possible for you to change the world for someone. My own life is proof we can use our own messy, broken, sea-sick, beautiful talents to move mountains.

I am currently living in Cambodia working with a faith-based, fair trade business that provides opportunities for men and women caught up in sex-work to make a new start through training, work, education, counseling, and healthy lifestyle courses, but Papua New Guinea will always be in my heart.

We will never be able to impact the world on our own. But, one thing is for sure, we will not do anything if we fail to move. "Liking" it on Facebook or even reading about issues won't solve problems.

So, go on.

Step out.

Take a risk.

Be who you were truly made to be.

Go.

Bring Life.

Hold nothing back. Love with everything.

Love in action. I guarantee it will transform a culture.

HOW TO GET INVOLVED

Go to Kapuna.org for contact information and volunteering at Kapuna Hospital.

If you want to donate to Kapuna, contact them for bank information at: kapunahosp@gmail.com.

Please specify what you want your donation to go for. Ex: Medical, Discipleship, Jadon's Toilet Project, etc.

Long-term opportunities—check out these amazing organizations:
- Mission Aviation Fellowship (MAF): www. maf.org.au
- Wycliffe Bible Translators (Affiliated with SIL International): www.wycliffe.org
- New Tribes Mission (NTM): ntm.org

Short-term opportunities:
- YWAM Medical Ships Australia: ywamships.org.au

To Impact from home check out Adriel Booker's blog: http://adrielbooker.com/love-a-mama/

And, as always, pray for Kapuna and Papua New Guinea: the people, the organizations, the students, the staff, the government, etc.

ACKNOWLEDGMENTS

More than anything, I know God directed my steps to write this book. I am so grateful for the opportunity to use my gift in writing to share the incredible story of this bush hospital and the people who went in obedience, changing the health care and development of a dense jungle location. Without God, there would be no story to tell.

I want to thank the Calvert and Petterson families, staff, volunteers, students, and patients at Kapuna Hospital for letting me tell their story. More than that, you made me your *wantok* and I am so blessed by you all. Also, thanks to Dr. Beth for being a good friend and the catalyst for me to connect. I am also thankful for my friends at YWAM Townsville who encouraged me and released me to do this book, especially Ryan and Adriel Booker. I know you all are as in love with Papua New Guinea as I am.

I am grateful to my parents for raising me with a love for the marginalized and a determination to pursue justice in many capacities. I am also grateful for the many missionaries with SIL, MAF, and New Tribes Missions who befriended me, flew me across the bush, and shared your lives with me; you are all so much a part of this story. I am grateful for all of my friends around the world who prayed for me, read my work, and gave me a place to live while I wrote. A special thanks to Darcy, Jay, and little Soraya Clark for sharing your family and home with me for so long.

Thanks to Dave Weitz who not only has supported me over the years but introduced me to the amazing staff at Aloha Publishing. My gratitude overflows for Hannah, Maryanna, and the team at Aloha Publishing for not only being amazing to work with, but for falling in love with Kapuna along with me. You have great vision, helping the whole product come together.

My supporters and home church, The Pursuit, are also in this. Your generosity has enabled me to work as a full-time volunteer. I seriously have the coolest life. You bought plane tickets, kept food in my belly, and are just amazing at encouraging me.

Big thanks to Gerald for encouraging me to not give up on the frustrating communication and transportation in the process of getting to Kapuna. Debbie, you are the reason I got a flight into the bush. You are so "useful" and "gorgeous."

Finally, I want to thank the people of PNG. No matter where I have been in your beautiful country, you have taken me into your hearts and made me *wantok*. I cannot begin to tell you how much you all have changed my heart and my life. You have an unquenchable strength and beauty.

ABOUT THE AUTHOR

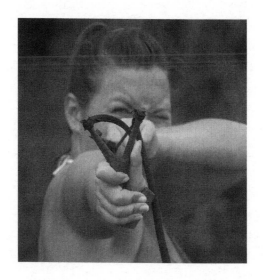

While she carries a US Passport, Erin Foley considers herself an international nomad, lover of all people and places. Studying journalism and photography at Hillsdale College in Michigan, USA, she graduated with a BA in Art in 2005. In 2011, she left the "American Dream" to pursue the best-life-ever as a full-time volunteer in Australia with shorter-term stints to Nicaragua, Papua New Guinea, East Timor, Spain and France. She is a stubborn middle-child who is slightly addicted to coffee, really wants a pet wombat, and wishes life was a musical.

She currently serves as a full-time volunteer in Cambodia with a faith-based organization established to offer men and women in the sex industry a fair-trade job, training, counseling, and healthy lifestyles.

Erin developed a strong sense of hatred toward injustice stemming from exposure to the third world and extreme poverty in her early childhood. Yet, stronger than her hatred toward injustice is her love of people, cultures, and travel. She desires to go deep, forging understanding, and build relationships through the process. She believes God does not want to change cultures but to redeem them, and so, she must act with His heart to see the bright spots He created in all groups of people.

Her aspiration: love would be the root of it all. Her writing is an expression of this love. She writes to call out the bright spots and encourage others to do the same. She does not believe in writing to gain acclaim or appease readers. She writes because she is passionate about using words to paint truth and take people on a journey; an instrument to always bless and handle each person's story in humility and as a precious gift.

Her life is completely wrecked for the ordinary. And, it really is an extraordinary life to live!

45156516R00155

Made in the USA
Charleston, SC
13 August 2015